SpringerBriefs in Statistics

JSS Research Series in Statistics

The current research of statistics in Japan has expanded in several directions in line with recent trends in academic activities in the area of statistics and statistical sciences over the globe. The core of these research activities in statistics in Japan has been the Japan Statistical Society (JSS). This society, the oldest and largest academic organization for statistics in Japan, was founded in 1931 by a handful of pioneer statisticians and economists and now has a history of about 80 years. Many distinguished scholars have been members, including the influential statistician Hirotugu Akaike, who was a past president of JSS, and the notable mathematician Kiyosi Itô, who was an earlier member of the Institute of Statistical Mathematics (ISM), which has been a closely related organization since the establishment of ISM. The society has two academic journals: the Journal of the Japan Statistical Society (English Series) and the Journal of the Japan Statistical Society (Japanese Series). The membership of JSS consists of researchers, teachers, and professional statisticians in many different fields including mathematics, statistics, engineering, medical sciences, government statistics, economics, business, psychology, education, and many other natural, biological, and social sciences. The JSS Series of Statistics aims to publish recent results of current research activities in the areas of statistics and statistical sciences in Japan that otherwise would not be available in English; they are complementary to the two JSS academic journals, both English and Japanese. Because the scope of a research paper in academic journals inevitably has become narrowly focused and condensed in recent years, this series is intended to fill the gap between academic research activities and the form of a single academic paper. The series will be of great interest to a wide audience of researchers, teachers, professional statisticians, and graduate students in many countries who are interested in statistics and statistical sciences, in statistical theory, and in various areas of statistical applications.

More information about this series at http://www.springer.com/series/13497

Achim Dörre · Takeshi Emura

Analysis of Doubly Truncated Data

An Introduction

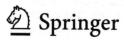 Springer

Achim Dörre
Department of Economics
University of Rostock
Rostock, Germany

Takeshi Emura
Graduate Institute of Statistics
National Central University
Taoyuan City, Taiwan

ISSN 2191-544X   ISSN 2191-5458   (electronic)
SpringerBriefs in Statistics
ISSN 2364-0057   ISSN 2364-0065   (electronic)
JSS Research Series in Statistics
ISBN 978-981-13-6240-8   ISBN 978-981-13-6241-5   (eBook)
https://doi.org/10.1007/978-981-13-6241-5

This Springer imprint is published by the registered company Springer Nature Singapore Pte Ltd.
The registered company address is: 152 Beach Road, #21-01/04 Gateway East, Singapore 189721, Singapore

Preface

This book provides fundamental ideas and statistical methodologies for analyzing *doubly truncated data*, and serves as an accessible introductory textbook for statistical analyses of doubly truncated data for students in statistics, mathematics and econometrics.

Scientific researchers may encounter difficulty to acquire samples whose measurements are outside specific ranges. Efron and Petrosian (1999, *JASA* 94: 824–34) provide an insightful example of *double-truncation*, where astronomical researchers cannot assess the luminosity of quasars if they are too dim (*left-truncation*) or too bright (*right-truncation*). In many scientific studies, samples may slip off from the data due to their measurements. The problem of double-truncation arises especially when researchers try to use field data or observational data to make inference on a population. *Double-truncation* may cause a systematic bias in the contents of data due to loss of information.

Although doubly truncated data are often observed in many fields of science, such as economics, medicine, engineering and so forth, there is so far no book that systematically presents the statistical methods needed for dealing with doubly truncated data. This book introduces readers to a variety of statistical methods for analyzing doubly truncated data, such as likelihood-based methods, Bayesian methods, nonparametric methods and linear regression methods. They can be used to analyze continuous data, especially lifetime data arising from biostatistics, economics and engineering. As truncation is a phenomenon that is often encountered in a variety of non-experimental studies, the methods presented in this book can be applied to many branches of science.

As the subtitle "An Introduction" suggests, we focus on basic methodologies and their mathematical foundations, rather than comprehensively reviewing all the existing methods. We try to offer clearer and more detailed explanations than those found in original articles. Consequently, the book may serve as a textbook especially suitable for master students majoring in statistics, mathematics, econometrics and other fields.

The book provides computer codes for most presented statistical methods to help readers analyze their data. The book can also serve as a research monograph, where each chapter can be read independently.

Rostock, Germany   Achim Dörre
Taoyuan City, Taiwan   Takeshi Emura

Acknowledgements

We thank the series editor, Dr. Shigeyuki Matsui for his valuable comments on this book.

The contents of the book have been presented in different places, including *CM Statistics 2013 conference* (in London, United Kingdom), *IMS-APRM 2014 conference* (in Taipei, Taiwan), *Complex time-to event data 2015* (in Louvain-La-Neuve, Belgium), *Statistical Week 2016* (in Augsburg, Germany), *Statistical Week 2017* (in Rostock, Germany), *CM Statistics 2018 conference* (in Pisa, Italy), a seminar in *National Chengchi University* (in 2013) and a seminar in *National Cheng Kung University* (in 2015). We thank all the organizers of the conferences and seminars as well as those who listened to our speeches and gave us valuable comments.

Achim Dörre thanks Gordon Frank for his prior contribution for the article Frank and Dörre [2017 *South African Statist J* 51(1): 1–18]. He also thanks Rafael Weißbach for constructive conversations on related topics. Finally, he thanks Ann-Josephine Thieme for many valuable discussions, support and perpetual motivation.

Takeshi Emura thanks Ya-Hsuan Hu for her prior contribution through the article of Hu and Emura [2015 *Computation Stat* 30 (4): 1199–229] and Yoshihiko Konno for his prior contribution through the article of Emura et al. [2017 *Stat Pap* 58 (3): 877–909]. Emura T. is financially supported by Ministry of Science and Technology, Taiwan (MOST 107-2118-M-008-003-MY3).

Contents

Abbreviations

AIC	Akaike Information Criterion
CI	Confidence Interval
i.n.i.d.	Independent but Not Identically Distributed
MCMC	Markov Chain Monte Carlo
MLE	Maximum Likelihood Estimator
NPMLE	Nonparametric Maximum Likelihood Estimator
NR	Newton–Raphson
R	A free software for statistical computing available from https://www.r-project.org/
SD	Standard Deviation
SE	Standard Error
SEF	Special Exponential Family

Notations

$a \in A$	An element a belonging to a set A
$\mathbf{a}^{\mathsf{T}}$	The transpose of a vector $\mathbf{a}$
$\mathrm{Bin}(n, p)$	Binomial distribution with size n and probability p
$\mathrm{E}(X)$	The expectation of a random variable X
$\mathrm{E}(X|A)$	The conditional expectation of a random variable X given an event A
$\mathbb{N}$	Natural numbers, i.e. $\mathbb{N} = \{1, 2, \ldots\}$
$\mathbb{N}_0$	Natural numbers including zero, i.e. $\mathbb{N}_0 = \{0, 1, 2, \ldots\}$
$N(0, 1)$	The standard normal distribution
$N(\mu, \sigma^2)$	Normal distribution with mean μ and variance σ^2
$N_k(\boldsymbol{\mu}, \Omega)$	k-dimensional multivariate normal distribution with mean $\boldsymbol{\mu}$ and covariance Ω
$I(\cdot)$	The indicator function: $I(A) = 1$ if A is true, or $I(A) = 0$ if A is false
$\mathrm{P}(A)$	The probability of an event A
$\mathrm{P}(A|B)$	The conditional probability of an event A given an event B
$\mathrm{Poi}(\lambda)$	Poisson distribution with intensity λ
$\mathbb{R}$	Real line or one-dimensional Euclidean space, i.e. $\mathbb{R} \equiv (-\infty, \infty)$
$\mathbb{R}^k$	A k-dimensional Euclidean space, e.g. $$\mathbb{R}^3 \equiv \mathbb{R} \times \mathbb{R} \times \mathbb{R} \equiv \{(x_1, x_2, x_3) : x_1 \in \mathbb{R}, x_2 \in \mathbb{R}, x_3 \in \mathbb{R}\}$$
$\mathbb{R}_{\geq 0}$	Non-negative real line, i.e. $\mathbb{R}_{\geq 0} \equiv [0, \infty)$
$\mathrm{tr}(\Omega)$	The trace of a square matrix Ω
$\mathrm{Unif}(a, b)$	Uniform distribution on an interval (a, b)
u_i or U_i	A left-truncation limit (after truncation)
u_i^* or U_i^*	A left-truncation limit (before truncation)
$\mathrm{Var}(X)$	The variance of a random variable X
v_i or V_i	A right-truncation limit (after truncation)
v_i^* or V_i^*	A right-truncation limit (before truncation)
$\Phi(.)$	The cumulative distribution function of $N(0, 1)$
$\phi(.)$	The probability density function of $N(0, 1)$
$\forall$	For any
$\xrightarrow{d}$ or $\xrightarrow{D}$	Convergence in distribution

$\xrightarrow{P}$	Convergence in probability
$\approx$	$x \approx y$ means x is approximately equal to y
$\sim$	$X \sim F$ means a random variable X follows a distribution F
$\equiv$ or $:=$	$x \equiv y$ means x is defined by y

Chapter 1
Introduction to Double-Truncation

Abstract This chapter introduces the basic terminologies and main themes of the book. We first illustrate the issues of double-truncation through real examples arising from economics, medicine and engineering. After discussing the issues of sampling bias due to double-truncation, we briefly review likelihood-based inference methods for doubly truncated data. We finally compare double-truncation with interval/right censoring.

Keywords Biased sampling · Lifetime data · Maximum likelihood estimation · Random double-truncation · Survival analysis · Truncated data

1.1 Doubly Truncated Data

In *simple random sampling*, an individual is selected randomly from the population of interest. This implies that individuals in the population are equally likely to be chosen by researchers. The dataset collected under simple random sampling provides unbiased information about the population. For instance, to estimate the mean lifetime of electric machines produced in a factory, one may randomly select machines and conduct a life testing experiment to measure the lifetimes of the machines. The sample average of the measured lifetimes provides an unbiased estimate of the population lifetime.

Truncation refers to a phenomenon that some individuals in the population have lower chance to be selected due to their too short or too long measurement. In this case, the probability that an individual is chosen from a population depends on its measurement. For instance, in many studies of lifetime, it may be too expensive or time-consuming to achieve simple random sampling from a target population. In particular, one cannot identify an individual whose lifetime is shorter or longer than a threshold, which is called *truncation limit*. In general, the value for the truncation limit varies with an individual. Whether an individual is selected into data is determined by the relationship between the measurement and its truncation limit.

Left-truncation is the most common type of truncation, where the data collection scheme tends to miss individuals with short measurement. For instance, if an electric machine has been broken and discarded before the initiation of life testing, the machine and its lifetime is said to be *left-truncated*. In this example, the time of the study initiation is defined as *left-truncation time* or *left-truncation limit*. Researchers obtain those individuals whose lifetime is longer than the left-truncation limit. Nevertheless, they wish to make inference on the population of all individuals without being influenced by the left-truncation. Left-truncation arises very commonly in biostatistics (Klein and Moeschberger 2003; Rodríguez-Girondo et al. 2018) and is often found in reliability theory (Kalbfleisch and Lawless 1992; Sect. 2.4 of Lawless 2003).

Right-truncation is another common type of truncation, where the data collection scheme tends to miss individuals with long lifetime. An individual is selected into the dataset if the lifetime is shorter than the *right-truncation limit*. A well-known example of right-truncation appears in the analysis of the incubation time of AIDS (Lagakos et al. 1998). A more recent example is found in the survival data for centenarians (Emura and Murotani 2015).

Double-truncation is a type of truncation where left-truncation and right-truncation occur simultaneously. For example, in astronomy, stellar objects in galaxies are undetected if they are too bright or too dim. Efron and Petrosian (1999) provide the case where quasars are observed only when their luminosity is between a lower detection limit and an upper detection limit. If the luminosity is too low or too high, it is undetected by astronomical instruments. This quasar example motivated the subsequent development for survival analysis with double-truncation, although luminosity is not *lifetime* in a literal sense. In the analysis of survival data, one obtains an individual if its lifetime falls between the left-truncation limit and right-truncation limit. In the following, we provide three data examples subject to double-truncation:

Example 1: The childhood cancer data of Moreira and de Uña-Álvarez (2010)
The term *childhood cancer* refers to cancers that occur between birth and 15 years of age. Moreira and de Uña-Álvarez (2010) provided a dataset on 406 children in North Portugal who were diagnosed with cancer during a 5-year recruitment period (between 1 January 1999 and 31 December 2003). The population of interest is a cohort of children in North Portugal. Children diagnosed before 1 January 1999 or after 31 December 2003 do not exist in the dataset, and hence, the data are doubly truncated.

Let y^* be the age at diagnosis of cancer for a randomly selected child from a population. The sample inclusion criterion is written as $u^* \leq y^* \leq v^*$, where u^* is the age on 1 January 1999 and $v^* = u^* + 5$ (years) is age on 31 December 2003 (Fig. 1.1). Thus, the left-truncation limit is u^* and right-truncation limit is v^*.

The dataset for Example 1 will be analyzed in Chap. 2.

Example 2: The German company data of Dörre (2017)
Data include German companies that were declared insolvent during the data collection period between 1 September 2013 and 31 March 2014 (Fig. 1.2). Let y^* be the lifespan of a randomly selected company from Germany (in years). However, the data do not have any information on companies who are declared insolvent

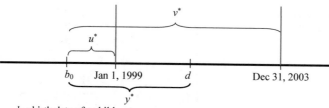

b_0 : birth date of a child

d : date of diagnosis (date of getting cancer)

y^*: age at diagnosis (age of getting cancer)

u^*: age on January 1, 1999 (u^* is negative for those born after Jan 1, 1999)

$v^* = u^* + 5$ (years): age on December 31, 2003

Fig. 1.1 The childhood cancer data of North Portugal (Moreira and de Uña-Álvarez 2010)

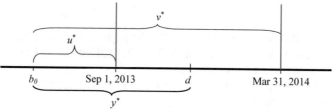

b_0 : date of founding of a company (*birth*)

d : date of insolvency (*death*)

y^*: lifespan of a company (in years)

u^*: age of a company on September 1, 2013 (in years)

$v^* = u^* + 7/12$: age of a company on March 31, 2014 (in years)

Fig. 1.2 The data on German companies (Dörre 2017)

outside this period. In particular, one cannot ascertain those companies whose business were initiated and then insolvent before the period (e.g. small companies). Also, one cannot ascertain those companies who continue their business beyond the period (e.g. large and stable companies). Formally, the sample inclusion criterion is written as $u^* \leq y^* \leq v^*$, where u^* is the age of a company on September 2013 and $v^* = u^* + 7/12$ for the 7-month period. Thus, the left-truncation limit is u^* and right-truncation limit is v^*. Restricting our attention to all companies formed after 2000, the dataset contains $n = 4139$ samples.

The dataset for Example 2 will be analyzed in Chaps. 3 and 5.

Example 3: The Equipment-S data of Ye and Tang (2016)

We introduce the equipment-S data given by Ye and Tang (2016). The data include failure times of units, called Equipment-S, and their installation dates that are varied from 1977 to 2012. The follow-up started at 1996 when the maintenance department realized the importance of collecting the data on Equipment-S. Hence a unit is

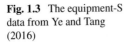

Fig. 1.3 The equipment-S data from Ye and Tang (2016)

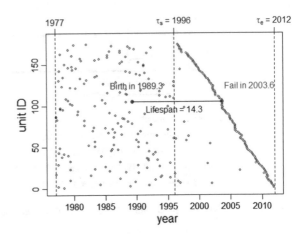

observed if it fails between 1996 and 2012. The population of interest is the set of all installed units. Unites failed before 1996 or after 2012 do not exist in the dataset, and hence, the data are doubly truncated.

Figure 1.3 is our attempt to mimic the data of Ye and Tang (2016) by reading off the numbers from their figure.

For instance, a unit has the year of installation in 1989.3 and the year of failure in 2003.6 (Fig. 1.3). Hence, the lifespan is $2003.6 - 1989.3 = 14.3$ (years). One can define the left-truncation limit u_i, the failure time y_i, and the right-truncation limit v_i in a similar fashion as Examples 1 and 2. Then, the data consist of (u_i, y_i, v_i) subject to $u_i \leq y_i \leq v_i$ for $i = 1, 2, \ldots, n$, where $n = 174$.

The dataset for Example 3 will be analyzed in Chap. 4.

Examples 1–3 have the same mathematical structure for truncation limits, namely, $v^* = u^* + d$ for some fixed constant $d > 0$. However, a practical distinction among them should be mentioned. In Example 1, the support of y^* is known to be [0, 15] since childhood cancers occur between birth and 15 years of age. The observed data mostly cover this range as $\min(y_i^*) = 0.0164$ and $\max(y_i^*) = 14.997$. This would be the case where nonparametric inference works well to estimate the distribution of y^*. However, in Examples 2 and 3, the upper bound of the support of y^* would be infinity since some company or machine can have a fairly long lifespan. The observed data may not cover the lifetime range. This would be the case where parametric inference provides more meaningful results than nonparametric inference by imposing a distributional assumption on the unobserved range of y^*.

In Examples 1–3, the distribution of truncation limits (u_i and v_i) is determined by the birth date on the calendar time axis. On the other hand, the distribution of the lifetime (y_i) is determined by the lifespan for an individual. Hence, two different time scales coexist; the calendar time scale and individual time scale. Chapter 3 provides more discussion on a *Lexis diagram* that simultaneously deals with the two time scales.

In Example 2 (the German company data), some covariates are obtained, which may be associated with the age of insolvency (Frank and Dörre 2017). This motivates us to consider a regression model (Chap. 5).

Notice that *censoring* is essentially different from truncation. In the presence of censoring, an individual's lifetime is known to be greater than a right-censoring limit, or less than a left-censoring limit. Thus, censoring yields incomplete ascertainment of lifetime while truncation yields incomplete ascertainment of samples. In Examples 1–3, individuals are not subject to censoring as their dates of failure are ascertained. If the sample inclusion criterion is the occurrence of failure, as in Examples 1–3, censoring usually does not arise.

1.2 Probability Models for Double-Truncation

To provide a probabilistic structure of double-truncation, we consider three random variables:

- y^*, a continuous lifetime having a density function f, namely $f(y) = d\mathrm{P}(y^* \leq y)/dy$,
- u^*, a left-truncation limit,
- v^*, a right-truncation limit.

Since doubly truncated data include those individuals satisfying $u^* \leq y^* \leq v^*$, we define the *inclusion probability* or *selection probability* defined as $\mathrm{P}(u^* \leq y^* \leq v^*)$. We typically assume independence between y^* and (u^*, v^*), namely,

$$\mathrm{P}(y^* \in A, (u^*, v^*) \in B) = \mathrm{P}(y^* \in A) \times \mathrm{P}((u^*, v^*) \in B)$$

for events A and B. An equivalent condition is

$$\mathrm{P}(y^* \leq y, u^* \leq u, v^* \leq v) = \mathrm{P}(y^* \leq y) \times \mathrm{P}(u^* \leq u, v^* \leq v) \quad \forall(y, u, v).$$

This assumption means that population lifetimes are not influenced by the truncation limits. However, the observed lifetimes in doubly truncated data are generally related to the observed truncation limits. This is because a shorter (longer) lifetime is accompanied by shorter (longer) range of truncation limits.

If one wishes to examine the independence assumption by a dataset, statistical tests can be performed. The test procedures examine a null hypothesis, called *quasi-independence* (Shen 2011). Quasi-independence is defined as

$$\mathrm{P}(y^* = y, u^* = u, v^* = v | u^* \leq y^* \leq v^*) = \frac{dF(y) \times dK(u, v)}{\iiint_{u \leq y \leq v} dF(y) \times dK(u, v)}, \quad (1.1)$$

for $\forall(y, u, v) \in S \equiv \{(u, y, v) : u \leq y \leq v\}$, where $F : \mathbb{R} \mapsto [0, 1]$ and $K : \mathbb{R}^2 \mapsto [0, 1]$ are distribution functions. Quasi-independence means that y^* and (u^*, v^*)

behave as independent variables within the set S. Clearly, the independence between y^* and (u^*, v^*) implies quasi-independence by setting $F(y) \equiv P(y^* \leq y)$ and $K(u, v) \equiv P(u^* \leq u, v^* \leq v)$.[1] Hence, the rejection of quasi-independence implies the rejection of the independence. However, the acceptance of quasi-independence does not imply the acceptance of the independence.

Efron and Petrosian (1999) and Martin and Betensky (2005) adopted a conditional version of Kendall's tau to assess the validity of quasi-independence using doubly truncated data. They provide two different tests for quasi-independence (a permutation test and a U-statistics test). Shen (2011) developed an alternative test by using a weighted log-rank statistic of Emura and Wang (2010).

Besides the independence assumption between y^* and (u^*, v^*), many practical models of double-truncation impose additional assumptions on the joint distribution of (u^*, v^*).

Random double-truncation means that u^* and v^* are continuous random variables having a joint density

$$k(u, v) = \frac{\partial^2}{\partial u \partial v} P(u^* \leq u, v^* \leq v).$$

Then, the inclusion probability is

$$P(u^* \leq y^* \leq v^*) = \iint_{u \leq v} \left[\int_u^v f(y) dy \right] k(u, v) du dv$$

$$= \int \left[\iint_{u \leq y \leq v} k(u, v) du dv \right] f(y) dy.$$

For instance, let $y^* \sim N(\mu, 1)$, $u^* \sim N(\mu_u, 1)$, and $v^* \sim N(\mu_v, 1)$ be independent random variables. Then, the inclusion probability is

$$P(u^* \leq y^* \leq v^*) = \int_{-\infty}^{\infty} \Phi(y - \mu_u)\{1 - \Phi(y - \mu_v)\}\phi(y - \mu) dy.$$

If $\mu_u = \mu - 0.91$ and $\mu_v = \mu + 0.91$, then $P(u^* \leq y^* \leq v^*) \approx 0.5$.

Fixed-length double-truncation is given by the relationship $v^* = u^* + d$, where d is a deterministic (non-random) value, and u^* is a continuous random variable having a density function

$$g(u) = \frac{d}{du} P(u^* \leq u).$$

---

[1]The event $\{y^* = y\}$ has a probability mass $P(y^* = y) = P(y^* \leq y) - P(y^* < y) = F(y) - F(y - dy) = dF(y)$. Similarly, the event $\{u^* = u, v^* = v\}$ has a probability mass $P(u^* = u, v^* = v) = dK(u, v)$. Thus, Eq. (1.1) holds under the independence.

Examples 1–3 are cases for fixed-length double-truncation. In these examples, the density of u^* describes the process of *birth*, and may have a known distribution type (e.g. the uniform distribution). The inclusion probability is

$$P(u^* \leq y^* \leq v^*) = \int \left[\int_u^{u+d} f(y) dy \right] g(u) du = \int \left[\int_{y-d}^y g(u) du \right] f(y) dy.$$

In Example 2 (the German company data), we obtain covariates that may be associated with the lifetime y^*. Let $\mathbf{z}^* = (z_1^*, \ldots, z_k^*)$ be a set of covariates that are independent of u^*. A linear model $y^* = \beta_1 z_1^* + \cdots + \beta_k z_k^* + \varepsilon^*$ can be considered, where $\beta = (\beta_1, \ldots, \beta_k)$ are regression coefficients and ε^* is an error term. In Example 2, the covariates are better treated as random variables (rather than the designed values). Accordingly, the inclusion probability is

$$P(u^* \leq y^* \leq v^*) = \int \int \left[\int_{y-d}^y g(u) du \right] f(y, \mathbf{z}) dy d\mathbf{z},$$

where $f(y, \mathbf{z})$ is the joint density of y^* and $\mathbf{z}^*$.

Chapter 2 considers parametric models on the distribution of y^* without assuming the distributions of u^* and v^*. Chapter 3 considers parametric models on both y^* and u^* under fixed-length double-truncation. Chapter 4 keeps the model nonparametric on all of y^*, u^* and v^*. Chapter 5 considers a linear model $y^* = \mathbf{z}^* \beta + \varepsilon^*$ without assuming the distributions of $\mathbf{z}^*$ and ε^*.

1.3 Truncation Bias

Let y_i^*, $i = 1, 2, \ldots$, be independent and identically distributed (i.i.d.) random variables following a density function f. Consider the case where simple random sampling can be adopted to collect data $\{y_i^*; i = 1, 2, \ldots N\}$ for a fixed number N. Then, the data provide unbiased information about the density f. For instance, the sample moment $\sum_{i=1}^N (y_i^*)^k / N$ is an unbiased estimator of the population moment $E[(y^*)^k] = \int y^k f(y) dy$ for $k = 1, 2, \ldots$.

Now we consider the case, where simple random sampling cannot be adopted due to double-truncation. Let u_i^* be a *left-truncation limit* and let v_i^* be a *right-truncation limit* associated with y_i^*. Under double-truncation, an individual becomes available only if $u_i^* \leq y_i^* \leq v_i^*$ holds. Then, the data consist of $\{(u_i, y_i, v_i); u_i \leq y_i \leq v_i, i = 1, 2, \ldots, n\}$. Such data are called *doubly truncated data*.

If naïve statistical methods for simple random sampling are applied to doubly truncated data, they yield biased information about f. For instance, the sample mean

$\bar{y} = \sum_{i=1}^{n} y_i/n$ gives a biased information about $E(y^*)$ since $\bar{y}$ is, in fact, estimating $E(y^*|u^* \leq y^* \leq v^*)$. Under random double-truncation,

$$E(y^*|u^* \leq y^* \leq v^*) = \frac{\iiint_{u \leq y \leq v} yf(y)k(u,v)dydudv}{\iiint_{u \leq y \leq v} f(y)k(u,v)dydudv}.$$

Under fixed-length double-truncation,

$$E(y^*|u^* \leq y^* \leq v^*) = \frac{\int \left[\int_u^{u+d} yf(y)dy\right]g(u)du}{\int \left[\int_u^{u+d} f(y)dy\right]g(u)du} = \frac{\int \left[\int_{y-d}^{y} g(u)du\right]yf(y)dy}{\int \left[\int_{y-d}^{y} g(u)du\right]f(y)dy}.$$

In general, $E(y^*) \neq E(y^*|u^* \leq y^* \leq v^*)$. An interesting exception is the uniform distribution for u^* in fixed-length double-truncation, whose density is defined as $g(u) = I(s \leq u \leq t)/(t-s)$. where $I(\cdot)$ is the indicator function. Then,

$$\int_{y-d}^{y} g(u)du = \frac{1}{t-s} \int_{\min[\max(s,y-d),t]}^{\min[\max(s,y),t]} 1 \cdot dy$$
$$= \frac{\min[\max(s,y),t] - \min[\max(s,y-d),t]}{t-s}.$$

If s is small enough and t is large enough, then $\int_{y-d}^{y} g(u)du = \frac{d}{t-s}$ for all y.[2] Then, $\sum_{i=1}^{n} y_i/n$ is unbiased for $E(y^*|u^* \leq y^* \leq v^*) = E(y^*)$. In general, however, analysis of doubly truncated data requires tailored methods for making unbiased statistical inference about the population density f.

1.4 Likelihood-Based Inference Under Double-Truncation

Likelihood-based analysis provides a systematic way of correcting bias due to truncation. As long as we construct a likelihood function by appropriately accounting for the probability distribution of observed data, unbiased inference for the population is feasible. Here, we formulate a likelihood function for making inference on the density f based on doubly truncated data $\{(u_i, y_i, v_i); u_i \leq y_i \leq v_i, i = 1, 2, \ldots, n\}$.

A general form of a likelihood function can be expressed as

$$L = \left[\prod_{i=1}^{n} P(u^* = u_i, y^* = y_i, v^* = v_i | u^* \leq y^* \leq v^*)\right] \times P(n),$$

---

[2]The value of $\min[\max(s, y), t] - \min[\max(s, y-d), t]$ has five different cases: (i) $y-d$ if $y-d < s < y$; (ii) 0 if $y < s$ or $y-d > t$; (iii) $t-y+d$ if $y-d < t < y$; (iv) $t-s$ if $y-d < s$ and $t < y-d$; (v) d if $s < y-d$ and $y < t$.

where $P(n)$ is the probability of observing the sample size n.

Due to the sampling scheme, the sample size n is generally a random variable and its distribution is linked to the random variables governing the truncation phenomenon. An inherent question is how to incorporate the randomness of n into the methodology. Essentially, n can be treated as part of the data, particularly because it carries information on the underlying distributions. In some settings, $P(n)$ contains information about f and greatly contributes to the efficiency of estimation. On the other hand, one usually needs a specific parametric model to derive the form of $P(n)$. However, since n determines the size of the remaining data vectors, it is not entirely trivial to properly include it in the likelihood function (see Chap. 3 for a discussion).

Consider the random vector (u_i^*, y_i^*, v_i^*) for each unit i in the population. The selection indicator for double-truncation is the function $\varphi(u_i^*, y_i^*, v_i^*) \equiv I(u_i^* \leq y_i^* \leq v_i^*)$, having values 0 and 1, such that the sample size is given as $n = \sum_{i=1}^{N} \varphi(u_i^*, y_i^*, v_i^*)$, where N denotes the size of the population. Evidently, n is random and its distribution depends on the joint distribution of (u_i^*, y_i^*, v_i^*). Related to this, there is a common probability $p = P[\varphi(u_i^*, y_i^*, v_i^*) = 1]$ of selecting a random unit i from the population, which shall be called selection or inclusion probability. For a given population size N, we see that n is binomially distributed as $Bin(N, p)$. This holds for parametric and nonparametric models. A key step to make use of this relation is to effectively determine or at least approximate the probability p for the underlying distributions.

Note that this view can be taken with either deterministic or random population size N. In the former case, the distribution of n depends on the discrete parameter N, which is often unknown and can lead to technical inconveniences. In the latter case, however, when N is treated random, it is possible to avoid the potential circumstances and derive the distribution of n without explicitly considering the realized value of N (see Chap. 3). Furthermore, it can be shown that incorporation of the randomness of n is usually not crucial, since its impact is asymptotically negligible in many cases; see Sanathanan (1972, 1977) and Lee and Berger (2001). For this reason, the randomness of n is not a major concern in many studies on double-truncation.

Hence, the term $P(n)$ is often ignored so that the likelihood function is defined conditional on the sample size

$$L_n = \left[\prod_{i=1}^{n} P(u^* = u_i, y^* = y_i, v^* = v_i | u^* \leq y^* \leq v^*) \right].$$

In the following, we separately discuss the likelihood function L_n for random double-truncation and fixed-length double-truncation.

1.4.1 Random Double-Truncation

We consider three random variables u_i^*, y_i^*, and v_i^*. The joint density of the observed data point (u_i, y_i, v_i) is

$$P(u^* = u_i, y^* = y_i, v^* = v_i | u^* \leq y^* \leq v^*) = \frac{P(u^* = u_i, y^* = y_i, v^* = v_i)}{P(u^* \leq y^* \leq v^*)}.$$

Combining all data points under random double-truncation, the likelihood function is defined as

$$L_n(f, k) \equiv \prod_{i=1}^{n} \frac{f(y_i)k(u_i, v_i)}{\iiint_{u \leq y \leq v} f(y)k(u, v)dydudv}.$$

Maximum likelihood estimation of f and k can be considered by maximizing $L_n(f, k)$ with respect to both f and k. However, if one is solely interested in estimation of f, the following arguments can simplify the problem.

By the law of probability, $P(A, B|C) = P(A|B, C)P(B|C)$, we write

$$P(u^* = u_i, y^* = y_i, v^* = v_i | u^* \leq y^* \leq v^*)$$
$$= P(y^* = y_i | u^* = u_i, v^* = v_i, u^* \leq y^* \leq v^*) \times P(u^* = u_i, v^* = v_i | u^* \leq y^* \leq v^*)$$
$$= P(y^* = y_i | u^* = u_i, v^* = v_i, u_i \leq y^* \leq v_i)$$
$$\times P(u^* = u_i, v^* = v_i, u_i \leq y^* \leq v_i | u^* \leq y^* \leq v^*)$$
$$= P(y^* = y_i | u_i \leq y^* \leq v_i) \times P(u^* = u_i, v^* = v_i, u_i \leq y^* \leq v_i | u^* \leq y^* \leq v^*)$$
$$= \frac{P(y^* = y_i)}{P(u_i \leq y^* \leq v_i)} \times \frac{P(u^* = u_i, v^* = v_i, u_i \leq y^* \leq v_i)}{P(u^* \leq y^* \leq v^*)},$$

where the second last equation follows due to the assumption of the independence between y^* and (u^*, v^*). Accordingly, one can decompose the likelihood function into two conditional likelihoods

$$L_n(f, k) = \prod_{i=1}^{n} \frac{f(y_i)}{\int_{u_i}^{v_i} f(y)dy} \times \prod_{i=1}^{n} \frac{\left[\int_{u_i}^{v_i} f(y)dy\right]k(u_i, v_i)}{\iiint_{u \leq y \leq v} f(y)k(u, v)dudydv}.$$

For making inference on the density f, Efron and Petrosian (1999) used the first part of the likelihood, namely

$$L_n(f) \equiv \prod_{i=1}^{n} P(y^* = y_i | u_i \leq y^* \leq v_i) = \prod_{i=1}^{n} \frac{f(y_i)}{\int_{u_i}^{v_i} f(y)dy}.$$

This is the likelihood that one can make statistical inference on f without modeling the distribution of truncation limits. The conditional likelihood $L_n(f)$ can be treated as the usual likelihood (Klein and Moeschberger 2003).

Under the nonparametric setting, Shen (2010) showed that the MLE based on $L_n(f)$ and the MLE based on $L_n(f, k)$ give an equivalent estimator for f. This remarkable property suggests that $L_n(f)$ contains sufficient information about f under the nonparametric setting.

1.4.2 Fixed-Length Double-Truncation

Recall that fixed-length double-truncation is given by the relationship $v^* = u^* + d$, where d is a deterministic (non-random) value, and u^* is a continuous random variable having a density function g. The density of the data point (u_i, y_i, v_i) is

$$P(u^* = u_i, y^* = y_i | u^* \leq y^* \leq u^* + d) = \frac{P(u^* = u_i, y^* = y_i)}{P(u^* \leq y^* \leq u^* + d)}$$

Combining all data points under fixed-length double-truncation, the likelihood function is defined as

$$L_n(f, g) \equiv \prod_{i=1}^{n} \frac{f(y_i)g(u_i)}{\int \left[\int_u^{u+d} f(y)dy \right] g(u)du}.$$

As previously demonstrated for the case of random double-truncation

$$P(u^* = u_i, y^* = y_i | u^* \leq y^* \leq u^* + d)$$
$$= P(y^* = y_i | u^* = u_i, u^* \leq y^* \leq u^* + d) \times P(u^* = u_i | u^* \leq y^* \leq u^* + d)$$
$$= P(y^* = y_i | u^* = u_i, u_i \leq y^* \leq u_i + d)$$
$$\quad \times P(u^* = u_i, u_i \leq y^* \leq u_i + d | u^* \leq y^* \leq u^* + d)$$
$$= P(y^* = y_i | u_i \leq y^* \leq u_i + d) \times P(u^* = u_i, u_i \leq y^* \leq u_i + d | u^* \leq y^* \leq u^* + d)$$
$$= \frac{P(y^* = y_i)}{P(u_i \leq y^* \leq u_i + d)} \times \frac{P(u^* = u_i, u_i \leq y^* \leq u_i + d)}{P(u^* \leq y^* \leq u^* + d)},$$

where the second last equation follows due to the assumption of the independence between y^* and u^*. Accordingly, one can decompose the likelihood function into two conditional likelihoods;

$$L_n(f, g) = \prod_{i=1}^{n} \frac{f(y_i)}{\int_{u_i}^{u_i+d} f(y)dy} \times \prod_{i=1}^{n} \frac{\left[\int_{u_i}^{u_i+d} f(y)dy \right] g(u_i)}{\int \left[\int_u^{u+d} f(y)dy \right] g(u)du}.$$

For making inference on the density f, one can use the conditional likelihood

$$L_n(f) \equiv \prod_{i=1}^{n} P(y^* = y_i | u_i \leq y^* \leq u_i + d) = \prod_{i=1}^{n} \frac{f(y_i)}{\int_{u_i}^{u_i+d} f(y)dy}.$$

This is the likelihood that can be used without specifying the distribution of the truncation time u^*.

1.4.3 Maximum Likelihood Estimation

We have seen that the conditional likelihood for f is written as

$$L_n(f) = \prod_{i=1}^{n} \frac{f(y_i)}{\int_{u_i}^{v_i} f(y)dy}.$$

This likelihood function can accommodate several different types of truncation. Fixed-length double-truncation corresponds to $v_i = u_i + d$, where $d > 0$ is a fixed number associated with the duration of sampling. Left-truncation corresponds to $v_i = \infty$, and right-truncation corresponds to $u_i = -\infty$. *Fixed double-truncation corresponds to $u_i = u_0$ and $v_i = v_0$, where $u_0 < v_0$ are fixed values.* Statistical inference under fixed double-truncation is extensively studied in the classical literature and summarized well in the book of Cohen (1991).

We provide a simple example to illustrate the likelihood function. Consider a dataset of $n = 4$, defines as $(u_1, y_1, v_1) = (0, 2, 3)$, $(u_2, y_2, v_2) = (2, 5, 8)$, $(u_3, y_3, v_3) = (5, 8, 9)$ and $(u_4, y_4, v_4) = (0, 1, 7)$. Then, the likelihood function is

$$L_n(f) = \frac{f(2)}{\int_0^3 f(y)dy} \times \frac{f(5)}{\int_2^8 f(y)dy} \times \frac{f(8)}{\int_5^9 f(y)dy} \times \frac{f(1)}{\int_0^7 f(y)dy}.$$

We shall demonstrate the computation of the MLE under a simple parametric model given by

$$f_\eta(y) = -\eta \exp(\eta y), \quad y > 0,$$

where $\eta < 0$ is an unknown parameter. Clearly, the model follows an exponential distribution with the mean $E_\eta(y^*) = -1/\eta$. This model turns out to be a special case of the special exponential family (Efron and Petrosian 1999; Emura and Hu 2015; Emura et al. 2017). Under this model, the log-likelihood is

$$\ell_{n=4}(\eta) = 4\log(-\eta) + 16\eta - \log(-e^{3\eta} + 1) - \log(-e^{8\eta} + e^{2\eta})$$
$$- \log(-e^{9\eta} + e^{5\eta}) - \log(-e^{7\eta} + 1).$$

If we maximize the log-likelihood numerically, we obtain the MLE $\hat{\eta} = -0.1099$. We also obtain the same result from the following codes with the R package *double.truncation* (Emura et al. 2019a):

```
library(double.truncation)
u.trunc=c(0,2,5,0)
y.trunc=c(2,5,8,1)
v.trunc=c(3,8,9,7)
PMLE.SEF1.negative(u.trunc,y.trunc,v.trunc,tau1=0)
```

The output is shown below:

```
$eta1
[1] -0.1098924

$SE1
[1] 0.3339333

$convergence
        logL            DF            AIC       No.of.iterations
    -6.167831      1.000000      14.335662           3.000000

$Score
[1] -1.600711e-10

$Hessian
[1] -8.967687
```

From the output, one can find the MLE $\hat{\eta} = -0.1098924$ at '\$eta1'. The package provides additional information besides the MLE, such as the standard error (SE) and the number of iterations. More details about the MLE are explained in Chap. 2.

If researchers do not wish to impose a particular parametric model on the population, a nonparametric approach can be considered. We shall introduce the *nonparametric MLE (NPMLE)* proposed by Efron and Petrosian (1999) under the dataset of $n = 4$. To define the NPMLE, we consider a discrete density function f that has positive probability masses at observed points of y_i's such that $f(1) + f(2) + f(5) + f(8) = 1$. Then, the likelihood is defined as

$$L_n(f) = \frac{f(2)}{f(1) + f(2)} \times \frac{f(5)}{f(2) + f(5) + f(8)} \times \frac{f(8)}{f(5) + f(8)} \times \frac{f(1)}{f(1) + f(2) + f(5)}.$$

The NPMLE is defined as a vector $\hat{\mathbf{f}} = (\hat{f}(1), \hat{f}(2), \hat{f}(5), \hat{f}(8))$ that maximizes the preceding equation subject to the constraint $f(1) + f(2) + f(5) + f(8) = 1$. The computing algorithm of the NPMLE and its theoretical properties are discussed in Chap. 4.

The NPMLEs of the distribution function and survival functions are $\hat{F}(y) = \sum_{y_i \leq y} \hat{f}(y_i)$ and $\hat{S}(y) = \sum_{y_i > y} \hat{f}(y_i)$, respectively. One may use the R package *double.truncation* (Emura et al. 2019a) to compute the NPMLEs $\hat{\mathbf{f}}$ and $\hat{F}(y)$.

There are different options to compute the SE of $\hat{F}(y)$ and the confidence interval of $F(y)$. Moreira and de Uña-Álvarez (2010) proposed a simple bootstrap method. Emura et al. (2015) used the asymptotic variance formula. The numerical performance of these two methods and the jackknife method are fairly comparable (Emura et al. 2015). The *double.truncation* package uses the asymptotic variance formula to compute the SE of $\hat{F}(y)$. Appendix A provides the explicit formula of the SE.

1.4.4   Other Estimation Methods

An alternative to the NPMLE is a kernel density estimation for f, which has been well-developed under double-truncation (Moreira and de Uña-Álvarez 2012; Moreira and Van Keilegom 2013; Moreira et al. 2014). The main advantage of the kernel estimators over the NPMLE is that it produces a smooth estimator of f. In fact, the NPMLE does not produce a meaningful estimator for f since it only gives us point masses. A kernel-smoothing estimation for the hazard function can also be considered by extending the approach of Weißbach et al. (2008) for right-censored data. The disadvantage of these kernel methods is the computational complexity of bandwidth selection. Another possibility is to apply cubic spline models that yield a smooth estimator for the density or hazard function (O'Sullivan 1998). The spline-based approaches appear to be a reasonable option but they have not been developed for analyzing doubly truncated data.

1.5   Relation to Censoring

There are several different types of missing data sampling schemes that resemble double-truncation.

Double-truncation is essentially different from *interval censoring*. Double-truncation produces biased sampling while interval censoring produces incomplete lifetimes (Commenges 2002; Collett 2003). In interval-censored data, event time is known to occur between a left-censoring limit l_i and a right-censoring limit r_i. Consequently, the likelihood function for interval-censored (IC) data is written as

$$L_n^{IC}(f) \equiv \prod_{i=1}^{n} \int_{l_i}^{r_i} f(y)dy.$$

Since the structures of $L_n(f)$ and $L_n^{IC}(f)$ are different, statistical methodologies for doubly truncated data are differently developed from those for interval-censored data.

Nonetheless, Turnbull (1976) considered both double-truncation and interval censoring under a nonparametric framework. *Doubly truncated and interval-censored (DTIC) data* consist of $\{\ (u_i, l_i, \ \ r_i, v_i);\ \ u_i \ \leq\ l_i\ \leq\ y_i\ \leq\ r_i\ \leq\ v_i,\ \ i\ = 1, 2, \ldots, n\ \}$ and the likelihood function is

$$L_n^{DTIC}(f) \equiv \prod_{i=1}^{n} \frac{\int_{l_i}^{r_i} f(y)dy}{\int_{u_i}^{v_i} f(y)dy}.$$

Turnbull (1976) developed a self-consistency algorithm to obtain the nonparametric MLE. Some additional work on doubly truncated and interval-censored data is referred to Shen (2013). The case of $v_i = \infty$ corresponds to left-truncated and interval-censored data, where the likelihood function can be applied to the analysis of the age-specific incidence of dementia (Joly et al. 1999).

Right-censored data is the most common type of data structures in survival analysis. Let y_i^* be the lifetime of interest and c_i be the random censoring time that is independent of y_i^*. Right-censored data consist of $(y_i, \ \delta_i)$ for each unit i in the population, where $y_i = \min(y_i^*, c_i)$, and $\delta_i = I(y_i^* \leq c_i)$. Right-censoring produces a complete case $\delta_i = 1$ (y_i^* is observable) or censored case $\delta_i = 0$ (y_i^* is only known to be greater than c_i). If the data do not involve any biased sampling mechanism, the likelihood function for right-censored (RC) data is written as

$$L_n^{RC}(f) \equiv \prod_{i=1}^{n} f(y_i)^{\delta_i} \left[\int_{y_i}^{\infty} f(y)dy \right]^{1-\delta_i}.$$

Again, the structures of $L_n(f)$ and $L_n^{RC}(f)$ are different.

Censoring can often be treated without explicitly modeling the censoring mechanism. In fact, the likelihood function $L_n^{RC}(f)$ contains all information about f under independent and non-informative censoring (Emura and Chen 2018). However, there may be no such simple consequence for double-truncation in general. In fact, the lifetime y^* and the truncation limits $(u^*, \ v^*)$ are inextricably connected to each other and thus carefully modeling the truncation limits is important. This may motivate us to adopt parametric models for both y^* and $(u^*, \ v^*)$, instead of simply using the conditional likelihood $L_n(f)$. This suggests that the full likelihood $L_n(f, k)$ may provide a more efficient estimator than the conditional likelihood $L_n(f)$ does. Overall, conditional likelihood approaches are adaptive to various types of regression models including the accelerated failure time model (Huang et al. 2019), Cox regression (Shen and Liu 2017), and transformation model (Shen and Liu 2019), with appropriate modifications.

This fact becomes even more fundamental when more expressive models such as regression models are considered. In those settings, estimating the specific parameters of interest hinges on the particular selection mechanism and its relation to the measured variates. In addition, measuring uncertainty of estimation, such as by standard errors, poses an additional challenge under truncation and uncertainty in any non-truncated model can be expected to be transported and perhaps even increased under truncation.

Interestingly, unlike the independent censoring assumption that cannot be verified, quasi-independence is a testable assumption with doubly truncated data (Efron and Petrosian 1999; Martin and Betensky 2005; Shen 2011). This encouraged the developments of models for *dependent truncation*. There are many statistical methods available for analyzing survival data with dependent left-truncation (e.g. Chaieb et al. 2006; Emura and Konno 2012a, b; Emura and Murotani 2015; Emura and Wang 2016; Emura and Pan 2017; Chiou et al. 2018a, b) and dependent right-truncation (e.g. Emura and Wang 2012). However, the literature is still scarce for doubly truncated data. While this book does not discuss this issue, analysis of dependently doubly truncated data is a promising area for future research.

Simultaneous occurrence of truncation and censoring is natural when observational data are collected over time. In the childhood cancer data, only truncation is acknowledged, but the occurrence of censoring by death might be possible. If a child dies before he/she gets cancer, the event time is censored by death. On the other hand, if a child dies after he/she gets cancer, both time-to-cancer and time-to-death are observable. Although statistical methods of bivariate event times are extensively developed by applying copula-based methods (Emura et al. 2019b), double-truncation has not been considered in these contexts. There seems to be a vast scope of this research area in general. In principle, all conventional models and methods for data analysis may be considered when data are subjected to truncation. In many cases, these considerations have brought valuable insight.

References

Chaieb LL, Rivest LP, Abdous B (2006) Estimating survival under a dependent truncation. Biometrika 93(3):655–669

Chiou SH, Austin MD, Qian J, Betensky RA (2018a). Transformation model estimation of survival under dependent truncation and independent censoring. Statist Methods Med Res, 0962280218817573

Chiou SH, Qian J, Mormino E, Betensky RA (2018b) Permutation tests for general dependent truncation. Comput Stat Data Anal 128:308–324

Cohen AC (1991) Truncated and censored samples. Marcel Dekker, New York

Collett D (2003) Modelling survival data in medical research, 2nd edn. CRC Press, London

Commenges D (2002) Inference for multi-state models from interval-censored data. Stat Methods Med Res 11:167–182

Dörre A (2017) Bayesian estimation of a lifetime distribution under double truncation caused by time-restricted data collection. Stat Pap https://doi.org/10.1007/s00362-017-0968-7

Efron B, Petrosian R (1999) Nonparametric methods for doubly truncated data. J Am Stat Assoc 94:824–834

Emura T, Chen YH (2018) Analysis of survival data with dependent censoring, copula-based approaches, JSS research series in statistics. Springer, Singapore

Emura T, Hu YH, Huang CY (2019a) Double.truncation: analysis of doubly-truncated data, CRAN

Emura T, Hu YH, Konno Y (2017) Asymptotic inference for maximum likelihood estimators under the special exponential family with double-truncation. Stat Pap 58(3):877–909

Emura T, Konno Y (2012a) Multivariate normal distribution approaches for dependently truncated data. Stat Pap 53:133–149

Emura T, Konno Y (2012b) A goodness-of-fit tests for parametric models based on dependently truncated data. Comput Stat Data Anal 56:2237–2250

Emura T, Konno Y, Michimae H (2015) Statistical inference based on the nonparametric maximum likelihood estimator under double-truncation. Lifetime Data Anal 21(3):397–418

Emura T, Matsui S, Rondeau V (2019b), Survival analysis with correlated endpoints, joint frailty-Copula models, JSS research series in statistics, Springer

Emura T, Murotani K (2015) An algorithm for estimating survival under a copula-based dependent truncation model. TEST 24(4):734–751

Emura T, Pan CH (2017) Parametric likelihood inference and goodness-of-fit for dependently left-truncated data, a copula-based approach. Stat Pap https://doi.org/10.1007/s00362-017-0947-z

Emura T, Wang W (2010) Testing quasi-independence for truncation data. J Multivar Anal 101:223–239

Emura T, Wang W (2012) Nonparametric maximum likelihood estimation for dependent truncation data based on copulas. J Multivar Anal 110:171–188

Emura T, Wang W (2016) Semiparametric inference for an accelerated failure time model with dependent truncation. Ann Inst Stat Math 68(5):1073–1094

Frank G, Dörre A (2017) Linear regression with randomly double-truncated data. S Afr Stat J 51(1):1–18

Hu YH, Emura T (2015) Maximum likelihood estimation for a special exponential family under random double-truncation. Comput Statistics 30(4):1199–1229

Huang CY, Tseng YK, Emura T (2019) Likelihood-based analysis of doubly-truncated data under the location-scale and AFT model (in revision). Comput Stat

Joly P, Letenneur L, Alioum A, Commenges D (1999) PHMPL: a computer program for hazard estimation using a penalized likelihood method with interval-censored and left-truncated data. Comput Methods Programs Biomed 60(3):225–231

Kalbfleisch JD, Lawless JF (1992) Some useful statistical methods for truncated data. J Qual Technol 24:145–152

Klein JP, Moeschberger ML (2003) Survival analysis techniques for censored and truncated data. Springer, New York

Lagakos SW, Barraj LM, De Gruttola V (1998) Non-parametric analysis of truncated survival data with application to AIDS. Biometrika 75:515–523

Lawless JF (2003) Statistical models and methods for lifetime data, 2nd edn. Wiley, Hoboken, New Jersey

Lee J, Berger JO (2001) Semiparametric bayesian analysis of selection models. J Am Stat Assoc 96:1397–1409

Martin EC, Betensky RA (2005) Testing quasi-independence of failure and truncation via conditional Kendall's Tau. J Am Stat Assoc 100:484–492

Moreira C, de Uña-Álvarez J (2010) Bootstrapping the NPMLE for doubly truncated data. J Nonparametr Stat 22:567–583

Moreira C, de Uña-Álvarez J, Van Keilegom I (2014) Goodness-of-fit tests for a semiparametric model under random double truncation. Comput Stat 29(5):1365–1379

Moreira C, de Uña-Álvarez J (2012) Kernel density estimation with doubly-truncated data. Electron J Stat 6:501–521

Moreira C, Van Keilegom I (2013) Bandwidth selection for kernel density estimation with doubly truncated data. Comput Stat Data Anal 61:107–123

O'Sullivan F (1998) Fast computation of fully automated log-density and log-hazard estimation. SIAM J Sci Stat Comput 9:363–379

Rodríguez-Girondo M, Deelen J, Slagboom EP, Houwing-Duistermaat JJ (2018) Survival analysis with delayed entry in selected families with application to human longevity. Stat Methods Med Res 27(3):933–954

Sanathanan L (1972) Estimating the size of a multinomial population. Ann Math

Sanathanan L (1977) Estimating the size of a truncated sample. J Am Stat Assoc 72:669–672

Shen PS (2010) Nonparametric analysis of doubly truncated data. Ann Inst Stat Math 62:835–853

Shen PS (2013) Regression analysis of interval censored and doubly truncated data with linear transformation models. Comput Stat 28(2):581–596

Shen PS (2011) Testing quasi-independence for doubly truncated data. J Nonparametr Stat 23(3):753–761

Shen PS, Liu Y (2017) Pseudo maximum likelihood estimation for the Cox model with doubly truncated data. Stat Pap https://doi.org/10.1007/s00362-016-0870-8

Shen PS, Liu Y (2019) Pseudo MLE for semiparametric transformation model with doubly truncated data, JKSS. https://doi.org/10.1016/j.jkss.2018.12.003

Turnbull BW (1976) The empirical distribution function with arbitrarily grouped, censored and truncated data. J R Stat Soc Series B (Methodological) 290–295

Ye ZS, Tang LC (2016) Augmenting the unreturned for filed data with information on returned failures only. Technometrics 58(4):513–523

Weißbach R, Pfahlberg A, Gefeller O (2008) Double-smoothing in kernel hazard rate estimation. Methods Inf Med 47(02):167–173

Chapter 2
Parametric Estimation Under Exponential Family

Abstract This chapter considers likelihood-based inference methods for doubly truncated samples under a class of models called the special exponential family (SEF). We introduce specific models in the SEF, and computational algorithms for maximum likelihood estimators (MLEs) under these models. We review the asymptotic theory for the MLE and then give the standard error and confidence interval. We also introduce an R package "double.truncation" (Emura et al, double.truncation: analysis of doubly-truncated data, CRAN 2019) that provides the computational programs to fit doubly truncated data to the models. Finally, we analyze a real dataset for illustration.

Keywords Exponential family · Maximum likelihood estimation · Newton–Raphson algorithm · Survival analysis · Truncated data

2.1 Introduction

Efron and Petrosian (1999) considered likelihood-based methods for fitting doubly truncated data to a class of models called the special exponential family (SEF). In this chapter, we introduce the SEF, and computational algorithms for obtaining maximum likelihood estimators (MLEs) under specific models from the SEF, which were previously developed by Efron and Petrosian (1999) and Hu and Emura (2015). We also review the asymptotic theory for the MLE (Emura et al. 2017), which produces the methods for computing the standard error (SE) and confidence interval (CI). For illustration, we apply the methods to analyze the childhood cancer dataset (Moreira and de Uña-Álvarez 2010).

To allow readers to apply the likelihood-based methods to doubly truncated data, we developed an R package *double.truncation* (Emura et al. 2019). The package automatically computes the MLE, SEs, and other useful quantities to assess the fit of the model. The main computational tool in the package is the Newton–Raphson algorithm where the initial values are carefully chosen so that the algorithm reaches the maximum of the likelihood function.

© The Author(s), under exclusive license to Springer Nature Singapore Pte Ltd. 2019
A. Dörre and T. Emura, *Analysis of Doubly Truncated Data*, JSS Research Series in Statistics, https://doi.org/10.1007/978-981-13-6241-5_2

This chapter is organized as follows. Section 2.2 defines the SEF. Section 2.3 constructs the likelihood function. Section 2.4 describes the Newton–Raphson algorithm. Section 2.5 introduces the asymptotic theory and computes the SE and CI. Section 2.6 introduces our R package for statistical computing. Section 2.7 analyzes the real dataset, and Section 2.8 concludes.

2.2 Special Exponential Family (SEF)

In this section, we first define the SEF, and then introduce specific models that belong to the SEF. We also introduce the basic properties of the models such as the parameter space, support, density, survival function and mode. Throughout, we use the notations $\mathbb{R} = (-\infty, \infty)$ for real line and $I(\cdot)$ for the indicator function.

Definition 1 *(SEF)* We assume that a random variable Y^* follows the k-dimensional SEF, which is a continuous distribution with a density

$$f_{\boldsymbol{\eta}}(y) = \exp\{\boldsymbol{\eta}^{\mathrm{T}} \cdot \mathbf{t}(y) - \varphi(\boldsymbol{\eta})\} I(y \in \mathrm{y}),$$

where $\boldsymbol{\eta} = (\eta_1, \eta_2, \ldots, \eta_k)^{\mathrm{T}} \in \Theta$, $\mathbf{t}(y) = (y, y^2, \ldots, y^k)^{\mathrm{T}}$, $\mathrm{y} \subset \mathbb{R}$ is the support of Y^*, $\Theta \subset \mathbb{R}^k$ is a parameter space, and $\varphi(\boldsymbol{\eta})$ is a normalizing factor.

The SEF is a special case of a k-dimensional exponential family. The parameter $\boldsymbol{\eta} = (\eta_1, \eta_2, \ldots, \eta_k)^{\mathrm{T}} \in \Theta$ is called the *natural parameter* and the parameter space Θ is called the *natural parameter space* (p. 24 of Lehmann and Casella 1998). For the density to be well-defined, a pair (y, Θ) should be chosen so that

$$\int_{\mathrm{y}} \exp\{\boldsymbol{\eta}^{\mathrm{T}} \cdot \mathbf{t}(y)\} dy < \infty \quad \text{for } \boldsymbol{\eta} \in \Theta. \tag{2.1}$$

Let τ_1 be the lower bound and τ_2 be the upper bound for the support of Y^* such that $-\infty < \tau_1 < \tau_2 < \infty$. The integral in Eq. (2.1) exists for any $\boldsymbol{\eta} \in \mathbb{R}^k$ under a bounded support $\mathrm{y} = [\tau_1, \tau_2]$. In this case, one can choose any parameter space for Θ. However, it is fruitful to consider unbounded supports $\mathrm{y} = [\tau_1, \infty)$, $\mathrm{y} = (-\infty, \tau_2]$, and $\mathrm{y} = \mathbb{R}$. In these cases, the existence of the integral in Eq. (2.1) has to be considered carefully.

Table 2.1 shows a variety of models produced by the SEF, including the exponential distribution and normal distribution. These models satisfy Eq. (2.1).

Table 2.1 Specific models included in the k-dimensional SEF

k	Constraint	Support	Mean	Mode	Type of distribution
1	$\eta_1 > 0$	$y = (-\infty, \tau_2]$	$\tau_2 - 1/\eta$	τ_2	J-shaped
1	$\eta_1 < 0$	$y = [\tau_1, \infty)$	$\tau_1 - 1/\eta$	τ_1	Exponential
1	$\eta_1 \neq 0$	$y = [\tau_1, \tau_2]$	$\dfrac{\tau_2 \exp(\eta \tau_2) - \tau_1 \exp(\eta \tau_1)}{\exp(\eta \tau_2) - \exp(\eta \tau_1)} - \dfrac{1}{\eta}$	τ_1 or τ_2	Truncated Exponential
1	$\eta_1 = 0$	$y = [\tau_1, \tau_2]$	$(\tau_1 + \tau_2)/2$	None	Uniform
2	$\eta_2 > 0$	$y = [\tau_1, \tau_2]$	No formula	τ_1 or τ_2	Convex
2	$\eta_2 < 0$	$y = (-\infty, \infty)$	$-\eta_1/2\eta_2$	$-\eta_1/2\eta_2$	Normal
3	$\eta_3 > 0$	$y = (-\infty, \tau_2]$	No formula	τ_2 or L_η	Truncated skewed normal
3	$\eta_3 < 0$	$y = [\tau_1, \infty)$	No formula	τ_1 or M_η	Truncated skewed normal

Note $L_\eta \equiv \dfrac{-\eta_2 - \sqrt{\eta_2^2 - 3\eta_1 \eta_3}}{3\eta_3}$ and $M_\eta \equiv \dfrac{-\eta_2 + \sqrt{\eta_2^2 - 3\eta_1 \eta_3}}{3\eta_3}$. These are defined for $\eta_2^2 - 3\eta_1 \eta_3 \geq 0$. If $\eta_2^2 - 3\eta_1 \eta_3 < 0$, the mode is τ_2 for $\eta_3 > 0$ and τ_1 for $\eta_3 < 0$

2.2.1 One-Parameter Models

We introduce three specific models in the SEF with $k = 1$, including the exponential distribution. Since the parameter is only η_1, we will simply denote the parameter as η.

First, consider the case $\eta > 0$. The parameter space of η is $\Theta = \{\eta : \eta > 0\} = (0, \infty)$. If we let τ_2 be the upper bound for the support of Y^*, then

$$f_\eta(y) = \eta \exp\{\eta(y - \tau_2)\}, \quad y \in y = (-\infty, \tau_2].$$

This is a well-defined density since $\varphi(\eta) = \log\left\{\int_{-\infty}^{\tau_2} \exp(\eta y) dy\right\} = -\log \eta + \eta \tau_2$ for all $\eta \in \Theta$. Figure 2.1 displays the density with $\eta = 0.5$ or 1.5 and $\tau_2 = 4$. The mode is τ_2 and the mean is $E_\eta(Y^*) = \tau_2 - 1/\eta$. The corresponding survival function is

$$S_\eta(y) = \int_y^{\tau_2} \eta \exp\{\eta(t - \tau_2)\} dt = 1 - \exp\{\eta(y - \tau_2)\}, \quad y < \tau_2,$$

and $S_\eta(y) = 0$ for $y \geq \tau_2$.

Next, consider the case $\eta < 0$. Accordingly, the parameter space of η is $\Theta = \{\eta : \eta < 0\} = (-\infty, 0)$. Then the density becomes

$$f_\eta(y) = -\eta \exp\{\eta(y - \tau_1)\}, \quad y \in y = [\tau_1, \infty).$$

Fig. 2.1 The density $f_\eta(y)$ of one-parameter models with parameter η. The mean of each model is indicated by the circle

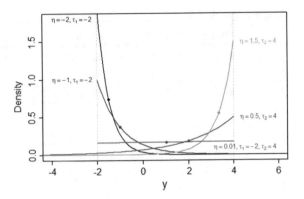

This distribution is a location-shifted exponential distribution. Figure 2.1 displays the density with $\eta = -2$ or -1 and $\tau_1 = -2$. The mode is τ_1 and the mean is $E_\eta(Y^*) = \tau_1 - 1/\eta$. The survival function is

$$S_\eta(y) = \int_y^\infty -\eta \exp\{\eta(t - \tau_1)\}dt = \exp\{\eta(y - \tau_1)\}, \quad y > \tau_1,$$

and $S_\eta(y) = 1$ for $y \leq \tau_1$.

Last, consider the case $-\infty < \eta < \infty$ so that the parameter space is $\Theta = \mathbb{R}$. Then, we must restrict the support by $y = [\tau_1, \tau_2]$ for $\tau_1 < \tau_2$. The density is

$$f_\eta(y) = \frac{\eta \exp(\eta y)}{\exp(\eta \tau_2) - \exp(\eta \tau_1)}, \quad \eta \neq 0, \quad \tau_1 \leq y \leq \tau_2.$$

Figure 2.1 displays the density with $\eta = 0.01$, $\tau_1 = -2$, and $\tau_2 = 4$. The mode is

$$\text{Mode} = \begin{cases} \tau_2 \text{ if } \eta > 0, \\ \tau_1 \text{ if } \eta < 0. \end{cases}$$

The mean is

$$E_\eta(Y^*) = \frac{\tau_2 \exp(\eta \tau_2) - \tau_1 \exp(\eta \tau_1)}{\exp(\eta \tau_2) - \exp(\eta \tau_1)} - \frac{1}{\eta}, \quad \eta \neq 0.$$

The survival function is

$$S_\eta(y) = \frac{\exp(\eta \tau_2) - \exp(\eta y)}{\exp(\eta \tau_2) - \exp(\eta \tau_1)}, \quad \eta \neq 0, \quad \tau_1 < y < \tau_2,$$

$S_\eta(y) = 1$ for $y \le \tau_1$ and $S_\eta(y) = 0$ for $y \ge \tau_2$.

The value $\eta = 0$ gives a uniform distribution $f_\eta(y) = 1/(\tau_2 - \tau_1)$, $\tau_1 \le y \le \tau_2$.

2.2.2 Two-Parameter Models

We introduce two specific models in the SEF with $k = 2$, including the normal distribution.

First, consider the case $\eta_2 < 0$ so that $\Theta = \{(\eta_1, \eta_2) : \eta_1 \in \mathbb{R}, \eta_2 < 0\}$. With $\mu = -\eta_1/2\eta_2$ and $\sigma^2 = -1/(2\eta_2)$, a normal distribution is obtained (see also Castillo 1994). The density is

$$f_\eta(y) = \frac{1}{\sqrt{\pi}} \exp\left\{ \eta_1 y + \eta_2 y^2 + \frac{\eta_1^2}{4\eta_2} + \frac{1}{2} \log(-\eta_2) \right\}, \quad y \in \mathsf{y} = \mathbb{R}.$$

Figure 2.2 displays the density. The survival function is

$$S_\eta(y) = \frac{1}{\sqrt{\pi}} \int_y^\infty \exp\left\{ \eta_1 t + \eta_2 t^2 + \frac{\eta_1^2}{4\eta_2} + \frac{1}{2} \log(-\eta_2) \right\} dt$$

$$= 1 - \Phi\left(\frac{y + \frac{\eta_1}{2\eta_2}}{\sqrt{\frac{-1}{2\eta_2}}} \right), \quad y \in \mathbb{R},$$

where $\Phi(.)$ is the cumulative distribution function of $N(0, 1)$.

Next, we consider the case $\eta_2 > 0$ so that $\Theta = \{(\eta_1, \eta_2) : \eta_1 \in \mathbb{R}, \eta_2 > 0\}$. Since the density is convex, the support must be bounded on a closed interval $[\tau_1, \tau_2]$. The density is

$$f_\eta(y) = \frac{\exp\left[\eta_2 \left(y + \frac{\eta_1}{2\eta_2} \right)^2 \right]}{\int_{\tau_1}^{\tau_2} \exp\left[\eta_2 \left(t + \frac{\eta_1}{2\eta_2} \right)^2 \right] dt}, \quad y \in \mathsf{y} = [\tau_1, \tau_2].$$

Fig. 2.2 The density $f_\eta(y)$ of the two-parameter models with parameters (η_1, η_2)

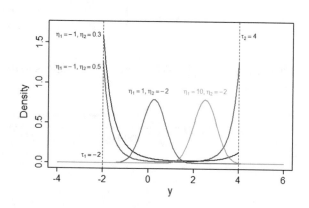

Since $\partial^2 \log f_\eta(y)/\partial y^2 = 2\eta_2 > 0$, the function $f_\eta(y)$ is strictly convex. If $-\eta_1/(2\eta_2) \in [\tau_1, \tau_2]$, then $f_\eta(y)$ has a minimum at $y = -\eta_1/(2\eta_2)$. Figure 2.2 displays the density with $\eta_1 = -1$, $\eta_2 = 0.3$ (or 0.5), $\tau_1 = -2$, and $\tau_2 = 4$. The mode of the density is

$$\text{Mode} = \begin{cases} \tau_1 \text{ if } \left|\tau_1 + \frac{\eta_1}{2\eta_2}\right| \geq \left|\tau_2 + \frac{\eta_1}{2\eta_2}\right|, \\ \tau_2 \text{ if } \left|\tau_1 + \frac{\eta_1}{2\eta_2}\right| < \left|\tau_2 + \frac{\eta_1}{2\eta_2}\right|. \end{cases}$$

The survival function is

$$S_\eta(y) = \frac{\int_y^{\tau_2} \exp\left[\eta_2\left(t + \frac{\eta_1}{2\eta_2}\right)^2\right] dt}{\int_{\tau_1}^{\tau_2} \exp\left[\eta_2\left(t + \frac{\eta_1}{2\eta_2}\right)^2\right] dt}, \quad \tau_1 < y < \tau_2,$$

$S_\eta(y) = 1$ for $y \leq \tau_1$ and $S_\eta(y) = 0$ for $y \geq \tau_2$.

2.2.3 Cubic Models

We introduce specific models in the SEF with $k = 3$ defined by the density

$$f_\eta(y) = \exp[\eta_1 y + \eta_2 y^2 + \eta_3 y^3 - \varphi(\eta)], \quad y \in y,$$

where the support y should be chosen so that $\varphi(\eta) = \log\left\{\int_y \exp(\eta_1 y + \eta_2 y^2 + \eta_3 y^3) dy\right\}$ exists. Note that $\partial f_\eta(y)/\partial y = (\eta_1 + 2\eta_2 y + 3\eta_3 y^2) f_\eta(y)$.

First, consider the case $\eta_3 > 0$ so that $\Theta = \{(\eta_1, \eta_2, \eta_3) : \eta_1 \in \mathbb{R}, \eta_2 \in \mathbb{R}, \eta_3 > 0\}$. Then, we must restrict the range of Y^* as $y = (-\infty, \tau_2]$. Figure 2.3 displays the density. If $\eta_2^2 - 3\eta_1\eta_3 < 0$, then the mode of the density is τ_2 since $\partial f_\eta(y)/\partial y > 0$. If $\eta_2^2 - 3\eta_1\eta_3 \geq 0$, the mode of the density is

$$\text{Mode} = \begin{cases} L_\eta \text{ if } f_\eta(\tau_2) \leq f_\eta(L_\eta), \\ \tau_2 \text{ if } f_\eta(\tau_2) > f_\eta(L_\eta), \end{cases}$$

where $L_\eta \equiv \frac{-\eta_2 - \sqrt{\eta_2^2 - 3\eta_1\eta_3}}{3\eta_3}$ is one of the solutions to $\partial f_\eta(y)/\partial y = 0$. The survival function is

$$S_\eta(y) = \frac{\int_y^{\tau_2} \exp(\eta_1 t + \eta_2 t^2 + \eta_3 t^3) dt}{\int_{-\infty}^{\tau_2} \exp(\eta_1 t + \eta_2 t^2 + \eta_3 t^3) dt}, \quad y < \tau_2,$$

Fig. 2.3 The density $f_\eta(y)$ of the cubic models with parameters (η_1, η_2, η_3)

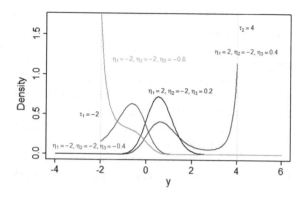

and $S_\eta(y) = 0$ for $y \geq \tau_2$.

Second, consider the case $\eta_3 < 0$ so that $\Theta = \{(\eta_1, \eta_2, \eta_3) : \eta_1 \in \mathbb{R}, \eta_2 \in \mathbb{R}, \eta_3 < 0\}$. Then, we must restrict the range of Y^* as $y = [\tau_1, \infty)$. Figure 2.3 displays the density. If $\eta_2^2 - 3\eta_1\eta_3 < 0$, then the mode of the density is τ_1 since $\partial f_\eta(y)/\partial y < 0$. If $\eta_2^2 - 3\eta_1\eta_3 \geq 0$, the mode of the density is

$$\text{Mode} = \begin{cases} M_\eta & \text{if } f_\eta(\tau_1) \leq f_\eta(M_\eta), \\ \tau_1 & \text{if } f_\eta(\tau_1) > f_\eta(M_\eta), \end{cases}$$

where $M_\eta \equiv \frac{-\eta_2 + \sqrt{\eta_2^2 - 3\eta_1\eta_3}}{3\eta_3}$ is one of the solutions to $\partial f_\eta(y)/\partial y = 0$. The survival function is

$$S_\eta(y) = \frac{\int_y^\infty \exp(\eta_1 t + \eta_2 t^2 + \eta_3 t^3)dt}{\int_{\tau_1}^\infty \exp(\eta_1 t + \eta_2 t^2 + \eta_3 t^3)dt}, \quad y > \tau_1,$$

and $S_\eta(y) = 1$ for $y \leq \tau_1$.

The cubic models yield a truncated skewed normal distribution, where η_3 determines the degree of skewness. For instance, Robertson and Allison (2012) fitted the US life table data with a truncated and skewed lifetime model that is similar to the cubic models. Knowing the asymmetry of the underlying data (i.e. skewness of the data) is essential for fitting parametric models to medical data (Mandrekar and Mandrekar 2003).

2.2.4 More Than Three Parameters

The SEF with more than three parameters may be useful to fit data having multiple peaks. The SEF with $k = 4$ ($k = 6$) can produce bimodal (trimodal) distributions. For instance, the parameters $\eta_1 = 0, \eta_2 = -0.8, \eta_3 = -0.1, \eta_4 = 1, \eta_5 = 0.1$, and $\eta_6 = -0.25$ yield a trimodal density in the range of $-2 < y < 2$. The SEF may serve as an alternative to finite mixture models, where two or more peaks are seen in the density. For applications of finite mixture models to survival analysis, see Chap. 10 of Everitt (2003) and McLachlan and McGiffin (1994).

We consider the case study of Matsui et al. (2005) who analyzed the incubation time for 76 patients with cadaveric dura mater-transmitted Creutzfeldt–Jakob disease reported in Japan. Data were right-truncated by the time at which the analysis was conducted; patients identified after November 2001 was excluded from the analysis. Their analysis revealed three peaks, short (1.4–6.2 years), medium (7.0–11.9 years) and long (12.9–17.6 years) incubation times. This might be a case where a trimodal distribution from the SEF with $k = 6$ is useful to fit the incubation time data.

2.3 Likelihood Function

We introduce the likelihood function under the SEF. Let $[u_i, v_i]$ be a truncation interval, where u_i is a left-truncation limit and v_i is a right-truncation limit. We consider estimation of $\boldsymbol{\eta}$ under the SEF when the random samples $y_1, y_2, \ldots, y_n$ are subject to double-truncation such that $u_i \leq y_i \leq v_i, i = 1, 2, \ldots, n$. The truncated density of Y^* within the interval $[u_i, v_i]$ is

$$f_i(y|\boldsymbol{\eta}) \equiv \frac{f_{\boldsymbol{\eta}}(y)}{F_i(\boldsymbol{\eta})} I(u_i \leq y \leq v_i)$$

where $F_i(\boldsymbol{\eta}) = \int_{u_i}^{v_i} f_{\boldsymbol{\eta}}(y) I(y \in y) dy$. Hence, the log-likelihood function is

$$\ell(\boldsymbol{\eta}) \equiv \log \left\{ \prod_{i=1}^{n} \frac{f_{\boldsymbol{\eta}}(y_i)}{F_i(\boldsymbol{\eta})} \right\} = \sum_{i=1}^{n} \{\log f_{\boldsymbol{\eta}}(y_i) - \log F_i(\boldsymbol{\eta})\}.$$

Under the SEF, the log-likelihood is computed as

$$\ell(\boldsymbol{\eta}) = \sum_{i=1}^{n} \boldsymbol{\eta}^{\mathrm{T}} \cdot \mathbf{t}(y_i) - \sum_{i=1}^{n} \log \left[\int_{u_i}^{v_i} I(y \in y) \exp\{\boldsymbol{\eta}^{\mathrm{T}} \cdot \mathbf{t}(y)\} dy \right].$$

Define $\hat{\boldsymbol{\eta}} = (\hat{\eta}_1, \hat{\eta}_2, \ldots, \hat{\eta}_k)^{\mathrm{T}}$ to be a solution to the score equations

$$\partial \ell(\boldsymbol{\eta}) / \partial \eta_j = 0, \quad j = 1, 2, \ldots, k, \tag{2.2}$$

where $\boldsymbol{\eta} = (\eta_1, \eta_2, \ldots, \eta_k)^{\mathrm{T}} \in \Theta$.

Theorem 1 *Suppose that Θ is open in $\mathbb{R}^k$. If the solution $\hat{\eta}$ to Eq. (2.2) exists, then it is the MLE, that is, $\ell(\hat{\eta}) \geq \ell(\eta)$ for any $\eta \in \Theta$.*

The proof of Theorem 1 is given in Emura et al. (2017) who utilized the concavity of $\ell(\eta)$.

2.3.1 One-Parameter Models

First, consider the case $\eta > 0$. As discussed previously, one needs to set the support $y = (-\infty, \tau_2]$. Whether a right-truncation limit v_i precedes the bound τ_2 influences the likelihood for a sample y_i. Consequently, the log-likelihood function is given by

$$\ell(\eta) = n \log \eta + \eta \sum_{i=1}^{n} y_i - \sum_{i=1}^{n} [\log\{\exp(\eta \min(v_i, \tau_2)) - \exp(\eta u_i)\}], \quad \eta > 0.$$
(2.3)

Hu and Emura (2015) used $\tau_2 = y_{(n)} \equiv \max_i(y_i)$ when maximizing Eq. (2.3). One can also use other plausible values for $\tau_2 > y_{(n)}$.

Next, consider the case $\eta < 0$. In this case, one needs to set the support $y = [\tau_1, \infty)$. Whether a left-truncation limit u_i exceeds the bound τ_1 influences the likelihood for a sample y_i. Consequently, the log-likelihood function is given by

$$\ell(\eta) = n \log(-\eta) + \eta \sum_{i=1}^{n} y_i - \sum_{i=1}^{n} [\log\{-\exp(\eta v_i) + \exp(\eta \max(u_i, \tau_1))\}], \quad \eta < 0.$$
(2.4)

Hu and Emura (2015) used $\tau_1 = y_{(1)} \equiv \min_i(y_i)$ when maximizing Eq. (2.4). One can also use other plausible values for $\tau_1 < y_{(1)}$.

Last, consider the case $-\infty < \eta < \infty$. In this case, one needs to set the support $y = [\tau_1, \tau_2]$ for $\tau_1 < \tau_2$. The log-likelihood function is given by

$$\ell(\eta) = \eta \sum_{i=1}^{n} y_i - \sum_{i=1}^{n} \log\left\{ \frac{\exp(\eta \min(v_i, \tau_2)) - \exp(\eta \max(u_i, \tau_1))}{\eta} \right\}, \quad \eta \neq 0.$$
(2.5)

One cannot rewrite the last term as $\log(A/\eta) = \log A - \log \eta$ since η is not always positive. Efron and Petrosian (1999) used $\tau_1 = y_{(1)}$ and $\tau_2 = y_{(n)}$. One can also use other plausible values for $\tau_1 < y_{(1)}$ and $\tau_2 > y_{(n)}$. If $\eta = 0$,

$$\ell(0) = -\sum_{i=1}^{n} \log[\min(v_i, \tau_2) - \max(u_i, \tau_1)].$$

When calculating the MLE, the case $\eta = 0$ can simply be ignored since the exact value $\eta = 0$ may not occur in numerical calculations of Eq. (2.5). The value $\ell(0)$ is useful when performing a likelihood ratio test for the null hypothesis $\eta = 0$.

2.3.2 Two-Parameter Models

First, consider the case $\eta_2 < 0$ so that $\Theta = \{(\eta_1, \eta_2) : \eta_1 \in \mathbb{R}, \eta_2 < 0\}$. Then, the log-likelihood function is given by

$$\ell(\eta) = \log L(\eta) = \sum_{i=1}^{n} \eta_1 y_i + \sum_{i=1}^{n} \eta_2 y_i^2 + \frac{n\eta_1^2}{4\eta_2} + \frac{n}{2} \log(-\eta_2) - \frac{n}{2} \log(\pi)$$
$$- \sum_{i=1}^{n} \log \left\{ \Phi \left(\frac{v_i + \frac{\eta_1}{2\eta_2}}{\sqrt{\frac{-1}{2\eta_2}}} \right) - \Phi \left(\frac{u_i + \frac{\eta_1}{2\eta_2}}{\sqrt{\frac{-1}{2\eta_2}}} \right) \right\}.$$

Next, we consider the case $\eta_2 > 0$ so that $\Theta = \{(\eta_1, \eta_2) : \eta_1 \in \mathbb{R}, \eta_2 > 0\}$. Then,

$$\ell(\eta) = \log L(\eta) = \sum_{i=1}^{n} \eta_1 \left(y_i + \frac{\eta_1}{2\eta_2} \right)^2 - \sum_{i=1}^{n} \log \left\{ \int_{\max(\tau_1, u_i)}^{\min(\tau_2, v_i)} \exp \left[\eta_1 \left(t + \frac{\eta_1}{2\eta_2} \right)^2 \right] dt \right\}.$$

2.3.3 Cubic Models

First, consider the case $\eta_3 > 0$. In this case, the parameter space is $\Theta = \{(\eta_1, \eta_2, \eta_3) : \eta_1 \in \mathbb{R}, \eta_2 \in \mathbb{R}, \eta_3 > 0\}$ and the support is $y = (-\infty, \tau_2]$. The log-likelihood function is

$$\ell(\eta) = \sum_{i=1}^{n} (\eta_1 y_i + \eta_2 y_i^2 + \eta_3 y_i^3) - \sum_{i=1}^{n} \log \left\{ \int_{u_i}^{\min(\tau_2, v_i)} \exp(\eta_1 t + \eta_2 t^2 + \eta_3 t^3) dt \right\}.$$

Hu and Emura (2015) used $\tau_2 = y_{(n)} \equiv \max_i(y_i)$ when maximizing the log-likelihood. One can also use other plausible values for $\tau_2 > y_{(n)}$.

Next, consider the case $\eta_3 < 0$. In this case, the parameter space is $\Theta = \{(\eta_1, \eta_2, \eta_3) : \eta_1 \in \mathbb{R}, \eta_2 \in \mathbb{R}, \eta_3 < 0\}$ and the support is $y = [\tau_1, \infty)$. The log-likelihood function is

$$\ell(\eta) = \sum_{i=1}^{n} (\eta_1 y_i + \eta_2 y_i^2 + \eta_3 y_i^3) - \sum_{i=1}^{n} \log \left\{ \int_{\max(\tau_1, u_i)}^{v_i} \exp(\eta_1 t + \eta_2 t^2 + \eta_3 t^3) dt \right\}.$$

Hu and Emura (2015) used $\tau_1 = y_{(1)} \equiv \min_i(y_i)$ when maximizing the log-likelihood. One can also use other plausible values for $\tau_1 < y_{(1)}$.

Last, we consider the case of $\eta_3 \in \mathbb{R}$. In this case, the parameter space is $\Theta = \mathbb{R}^3$, and the support is $y = [\tau_1, \tau_2]$. The log-likelihood function is

$$\ell(\boldsymbol{\eta}) = \sum_{i=1}^{n} (\eta_1 y_i + \eta_2 y_i^2 + \eta_3 y_i^3) - \sum_{i=1}^{n} \log \left\{ \int_{\max(\tau_1, u_i)}^{\min(\tau_2, v_i)} \exp(\eta_1 t + \eta_2 t^2 + \eta_3 t^3) dt \right\}.$$

Efron and Petrosian (1999) used $\tau_1 = y_{(1)}$ and $\tau_2 = y_{(n)}$. One can also use other plausible values for $\tau_1 < y_{(1)}$ and $\tau_2 > y_{(n)}$.

One potential concern for the cubic models is the unstability of the MLE due to the rich parameter space. In fact, the mean squared error for estimating η_1 and η_2 is remarkably larger under the cubic models than the mean squared error for estimating the same parameters under the two-parameter models with given $\eta_3 = 0$. Obviously, this concern is even more serious for the SEF with more than three parameters.

2.4 The Newton–Raphson Algorithm

Efron and Petrosian (1999), Hu and Emura (2015) and Emura et al. (2017) suggested using the Newton–Raphson (NR) algorithm to maximize the log-likelihood under the SEF. The NR algorithm is an iteration algorithm that employs the first- and second-order derivatives of the log-likelihood. In the R package *double.truncation* (Emura et al. 2019), the MLE is computed by the NR algorithm. This section provides the detailed implementation of the NR algorithms.

2.4.1 One-Parameter Models

For the case $\eta > 0$, the first- and second-order derivatives of the log-likelihood are

$$\frac{\partial}{\partial \eta} \ell(\eta) = \frac{n}{\eta} + \sum_{i=1}^{n} y_i - \sum_{i=1}^{n} \left\{ \frac{\min(v_i, \tau_2) \exp(\eta \min(v_i, \tau_2)) - u_i \exp(\eta u_i)}{\exp(\eta \min(v_i, \tau_2)) - \exp(\eta u_i)} \right\},$$

$$\frac{\partial^2}{\partial \eta^2} \ell(\eta) = -\frac{n}{\eta^2} - \sum_{i=1}^{n} \left[\frac{\{\min(v_i, \tau_2)\}^2 \exp(\eta \min(v_i, \tau_2)) - u_i^2 \exp(\eta u_i)}{\exp(\eta \min(v_i, \tau_2)) - \exp(\eta u_i)} \right]$$
$$+ \sum_{i=1}^{n} \left\{ \frac{\min(v_i, \tau_2) \exp(\eta \min(v_i, \tau_2)) - u_i \exp(\eta u_i)}{\exp(\eta \min(v_i, \tau_2)) - \exp(\eta u_i)} \right\}^2.$$

Similarly, for the case $\eta < 0$, one has

$$\frac{\partial}{\partial \eta}\ell(\eta) = \frac{n}{\eta} + \sum_{i=1}^{n} y_i - \sum_{i=1}^{n} \left\{ \frac{-v_i \exp(\eta v_i) + u_i \exp(\eta \max(u_i, \tau_1))}{-\exp(\eta v_i) + \exp(\eta u_i)} \right\},$$

$$\frac{\partial^2}{\partial \eta^2}\ell(\eta) = -\frac{n}{\eta^2} - \sum_{i=1}^{n} \left[\frac{-v_i^2 \exp(\eta v_i) + \{\max(u_i, \tau_1)\}^2 \exp(\eta \max(u_i, \tau_1))}{-\exp(\eta v_i) + \exp(\eta \max(u_i, \tau_1))} \right]$$

$$+ \sum_{i=1}^{n} \left\{ \frac{-v_i \exp(\eta v_i) + \max(u_i, \tau_1) \exp(\eta \max(u_i, \tau_1))}{-\exp(\eta v_i) + \exp(\eta \max(u_i, \tau_1))} \right\}^2.$$

For the case $\eta \in \mathbb{R}$, one has

$$\frac{\partial}{\partial \eta}\ell(\eta) = \frac{n}{\eta} + \sum_{i=1}^{n} y_i - \sum_{i=1}^{n} \left\{ \frac{\min(v_i, \tau_2) \exp(\eta \min(v_i, \tau_2)) - \max(u_i, \tau_1) \exp(\eta \max(u_i, \tau_1))}{\exp(\eta \min(v_i, \tau_2)) - \exp(\eta \max(u_i, \tau_1))} \right\},$$

$$\frac{\partial^2}{\partial \eta^2}\ell(\eta) = -\frac{n}{\eta^2} - \sum_{i=1}^{n} \left[\frac{\{\min(v_i, \tau_2)\}^2 \exp(\eta \min(v_i, \tau_2)) - \{\max(u_i, \tau_1)\}^2 \exp(\eta \max(u_i, \tau_1))}{\exp(\eta \min(v_i, \tau_2)) - \exp(\eta \max(u_i, \tau_1))} \right]$$

$$+ \sum_{i=1}^{n} \left\{ \frac{\min(v_i, \tau_2) \exp(\eta \min(v_i, \tau_2)) - \max(u_i, \tau_1) \exp(\eta \max(u_i, \tau_1))}{\exp(\eta \min(v_i, \tau_2)) - \exp(\eta \max(u_i, \tau_1))} \right\}^2,$$

for $\eta \neq 0$. In all the three cases, one can obtain the MLE of η by the NR algorithm. At each iteration, we obtain the updated parameter estimate

$$\eta^{(t+1)} = \eta^{(t)} - S(\eta)/\{\partial S(\eta)/\partial \eta\}|_{\eta=\eta^{(t)}},$$

for $t = 0, 1, 2, \ldots$, where $S(\eta) \equiv \partial \ell(\eta)/\partial \eta$ is the score function. The iteration continues until convergence, i.e. until $\left|\eta^{(t+1)} - \eta^{(t)}\right| < \varepsilon$ for some small $\varepsilon > 0$. Let $\bar{y} \equiv \sum_{i=1}^{n} y_i/n$ be the sample mean. For the case $\eta < 0$, we suggest the initial values $\eta^{(0)} \equiv 1/(\tau_1 - \bar{y})$ according to $E_\eta(Y^*) = \tau_1 - 1/\eta$. For the case $\eta > 0$, we suggest $\eta^{(0)} \equiv 1/(\tau_2 - \bar{y})$. For the case of $\eta \in \mathbb{R}$, we suggest $\eta^{(0)} \equiv 1/\{(\tau_1 + \tau_2)/2 - \bar{y}\}$.

2.4.2 Two-Parameter Models

We shall consider the case $\eta_2 < 0$ so that $\Theta = \{(\eta_1, \eta_2) : \eta_1 \in \mathbb{R}, \eta_2 < 0\}$. One can obtain the MLE by a two-dimensional NR algorithm. For $t = 0, 1, 2, \ldots$, the $(t+1)$th step of the iteration is

$$\begin{bmatrix} \eta_1^{(t+1)} \\ \eta_2^{(t+1)} \end{bmatrix} = \begin{bmatrix} \eta_1^{(t)} \\ \eta_2^{(t)} \end{bmatrix} - H^{-1}(\eta_1^{(t)}, \eta_2^{(t)}) \begin{bmatrix} S_1(\eta_1^{(t)}, \eta_2^{(t)}) \\ S_2(\eta_1^{(t)}, \eta_2^{(t)}) \end{bmatrix},$$

where $S_1(\eta_1, \eta_2) \equiv \partial \ell(\eta_1, \eta_2)/\partial \eta_1$ and $S_2(\eta_1, \eta_2) \equiv \partial \ell(\eta_1, \eta_2)/\partial \eta_2$ are the score function and

$$H(\eta_1, \eta_2) \equiv \left[\begin{array}{cc} \frac{\partial^2}{\partial \eta_1^2} \ell(\eta_1, \eta_2) & \frac{\partial^2}{\partial \eta_1 \partial \eta_2} \ell(\eta_1, \eta_2) \\ \frac{\partial^2}{\partial \eta_1 \partial \eta_2} \ell(\eta_1, \eta_2) & \frac{\partial^2}{\partial \eta_2^2} \ell(\eta_1, \eta_2) \end{array} \right].$$

is the Hessian matrix. Appendix B provides the explicit formulas for the score function and Hessian matrix. The iteration continues until convergence, i.e. until $\left| \eta_j^{(t+1)} - \eta_j^{(t)} \right| < \varepsilon \ \forall j$ for some small $\varepsilon > 0$. By the relationship $(\eta_1, \eta_2) = (\mu/\sigma^2, -1/2\sigma^2)$, we suggest data-driven initial values $(\eta_1^{(0)}, \eta_2^{(0)}) \equiv (\bar{y}/s^2, -1/2s^2)$, where $s^2 \equiv \sum_i (y_i - \bar{y})^2/(n-1)$.

2.4.3 Cubic Models

Since the NR algorithms are similar for the three cases ($\eta_3 > 0$, $\eta_3 < 0$, and $\eta_3 \in \mathbb{R}$), we only present the case of $\eta_3 \in \mathbb{R}$, where support of Y^* is a fixed interval $y = [\tau_1, \tau_2]$. For $\boldsymbol{\eta} = (\eta_1, \eta_2, \eta_3)^{\mathrm{T}}$, we define

$$E_i^k(\boldsymbol{\eta}) = \int_{\max(\tau_1, u_i)}^{\min(\tau_2, v_i)} y^k \exp(\eta_1 y + \eta_2 y^2 + \eta_3 y^3) dy, \quad k = 0, 1, \ldots, 6.$$

Since $E_i^k(\boldsymbol{\eta})$ does not have a closed-form expression, we shall apply a numerical integration routine (e.g. the *integrate* function in R). The first-order derivatives of the log-likelihood are

$$\frac{\partial}{\partial \eta_k} \ell(\boldsymbol{\eta}) = \sum_{i=1}^{n} \{y_i^k - E_i^k(\boldsymbol{\eta})/E_i^0(\boldsymbol{\eta})\}, \quad k = 1, 2, 3.$$

The second-order derivatives of the log-likelihood are

$$\frac{\partial^2}{\partial \eta_1^2} \ell(\boldsymbol{\eta}) = \sum_{i=1}^{n} [-E_i^2(\boldsymbol{\eta})/E_i^0(\boldsymbol{\eta}) + \{E_i^1(\boldsymbol{\eta})/E_i^0(\boldsymbol{\eta})\}^2],$$

$$\frac{\partial^2}{\partial \eta_2^2} \ell(\boldsymbol{\eta}) = \sum_{i=1}^{n} [-E_i^4(\boldsymbol{\eta})/E_i^0(\boldsymbol{\eta}) + \{E_i^2(\boldsymbol{\eta})/E_i^0(\boldsymbol{\eta})\}^2],$$

$$\frac{\partial^2}{\partial \eta_3^2} \ell(\boldsymbol{\eta}) = \sum_{i=1}^{n} [-E_i^6(\boldsymbol{\eta})/E_i^0(\boldsymbol{\eta}) + \{E_i^3(\boldsymbol{\eta})/E_i^0(\boldsymbol{\eta})\}^2],$$

$$\frac{\partial^2}{\partial \eta_2 \partial \eta_1} \ell(\boldsymbol{\eta}) = \sum_{i=1}^{n} [-E_i^3(\boldsymbol{\eta})/E_i^0(\boldsymbol{\eta}) + \{E_i^2(\boldsymbol{\eta})/E_i^0(\boldsymbol{\eta})\}\{E_i^1(\boldsymbol{\eta})/E_i^0(\boldsymbol{\eta})\}],$$

$$\frac{\partial^2}{\partial \eta_3 \partial \eta_1} \ell(\boldsymbol{\eta}) = \sum_{i=1}^{n} [-E_i^4(\boldsymbol{\eta})/E_i^0(\boldsymbol{\eta}) + \{E_i^3(\boldsymbol{\eta})/E_i^0(\boldsymbol{\eta})\}\{E_i^1(\boldsymbol{\eta})/E_i^0(\boldsymbol{\eta})\}],$$

$$\frac{\partial^2}{\partial \eta_3 \partial \eta_2} \ell(\boldsymbol{\eta}) = \sum_{i=1}^{n} [-E_i^5(\boldsymbol{\eta})/E_i^0(\boldsymbol{\eta}) + \{E_i^3(\boldsymbol{\eta})/E_i^0(\boldsymbol{\eta})\}\{E_i^2(\boldsymbol{\eta})/E_i^0(\boldsymbol{\eta})\}].$$

One can maximize the log-likelihood function by a three-dimensional NR algorithm. At each iteration, we update the parameters by

$$\begin{bmatrix} \eta_1^{(t+1)} \\ \eta_2^{(t+1)} \\ \eta_3^{(t+1)} \end{bmatrix} = \begin{bmatrix} \eta_1^{(t)} \\ \eta_2^{(t)} \\ \eta_3^{(t)} \end{bmatrix} - H^{-1}(\eta_1^{(t)}, \eta_2^{(t)}, \eta_3^{(t)}) \begin{bmatrix} S_1(\eta_1^{(t)}, \eta_2^{(t)}, \eta_3^{(t)}) \\ S_2(\eta_1^{(t)}, \eta_2^{(t)}, \eta_3^{(t)}) \\ S_3(\eta_1^{(t)}, \eta_2^{(t)}, \eta_3^{(t)}) \end{bmatrix}, \qquad (2.6)$$

$t = 0, 1, 2, \ldots,$ where $S_j(\eta_1, \eta_2, \eta_3) \equiv \partial \ell(\eta_1, \eta_2, \eta_3)/\partial \eta_j$ is the score function for $j = 1, 2,$ and $3,$ and

$$H(\boldsymbol{\eta}) \equiv \begin{bmatrix} \frac{\partial^2}{\partial \eta_1^2}\ell(\boldsymbol{\eta}) & \frac{\partial^2}{\partial \eta_1 \partial \eta_2}\ell(\boldsymbol{\eta}) & \frac{\partial^2}{\partial \eta_1 \partial \eta_3}\ell(\boldsymbol{\eta}) \\ \frac{\partial^2}{\partial \eta_2 \partial \eta_1}\ell(\boldsymbol{\eta}) & \frac{\partial^2}{\partial \eta_2^2}\ell(\boldsymbol{\eta}) & \frac{\partial^2}{\partial \eta_2 \partial \eta_3}\ell(\boldsymbol{\eta}) \\ \frac{\partial^2}{\partial \eta_3 \partial \eta_1}\ell(\boldsymbol{\eta}) & \frac{\partial^2}{\partial \eta_3 \partial \eta_2}\ell(\boldsymbol{\eta}) & \frac{\partial^2}{\partial \eta_3^2}\ell(\boldsymbol{\eta}) \end{bmatrix}$$

is the Hessian matrix. The iteration continues until convergence, i.e. until $\left| \eta_j^{(t+1)} - \eta_j^{(t)} \right| < \varepsilon \; \forall j$ for some small $\varepsilon > 0$.

It is well-known that the Newton–Raphson algorithm is sensitive to the initial values, especially in estimating three or more parameters (Knight 2000). To stabilize the algorithm, one may add random noises to the initial values. This scheme is called the *randomized NR algorithm* (Hu and Emura 2015) that has been applied to various models for survival data with many parameters (Emura and Pan 2017; Shih and Emura 2018; He and Emura 2019; Huang et al. 2019).

Randomized Newton–Raphson (RNR) algorithm

Let D_1, D_2, D_3, d_1 and d_2 be some positive tuning parameters.

Step 1. Choose the initial value $(\eta_1^{(0)}, \eta_2^{(0)}, \eta_3^{(0)}) \equiv (\bar{y}/s^2, -1/2s^2, 0)$.

Step 2. For $t = 0, 1, 2, \ldots,$ continue the iteration of Eq. (2.6) until convergence, i.e., until $\left| \eta_j^{(t+1)} - \eta_j^{(t)} \right| < \varepsilon \; \forall j$ and for some small $\varepsilon > 0$. Then $(\eta_1^{(t+1)}, \eta_2^{(t+1)}, \eta_3^{(t+1)})$ is the MLE.

Step 3. If $\left| \eta_1^{(t+1)} - \eta_1^{(t)} \right| > D_1,$ $\left| \eta_2^{(t+1)} - \eta_2^{(t)} \right| > D_2$ or $\left| \eta_3^{(t+1)} - \eta_3^{(t)} \right| > D_3$ occurs during the iterations, stop the algorithm. Replace $(\eta_1^{(0)}, \eta_2^{(0)}, \eta_3^{(0)})$ with $(\eta_1^{(0)} + e_1, \eta_2^{(0)} + e_2, \eta_3^{(0)}),$ where $e_1 \sim Unif(-d_1, d_1)$ and $e_2 \sim Unif(-d_2, d_2),$ and then return to Step 1.

2.5 Asymptotic Theory

The previous section focuses on the computation of $\hat{\boldsymbol{\eta}} = (\hat{\eta}_1, \hat{\eta}_2, \ldots, \hat{\eta}_k)$ under the SEF. This section discusses some asymptotic (large sample) theory, where the distribution of $\hat{\boldsymbol{\eta}} = (\hat{\eta}_1, \hat{\eta}_2, \ldots, \hat{\eta}_k)$ is approximated by a multivariate normal distribution with large n. Such an approximation is useful to derive the SE and CI.

Obviously, the major tool of asymptotic theory is the central limit theorem (CLT), i.e. the sum of independent random variables converges in distribution to a normal distribution (Lehmann 2004). To apply the CLT to doubly truncated samples, a technical issue is a treatment of non-identically distributed samples, as the sequence of random samples $y_1, y_2, \ldots, y_n$ are independent but not identically distributed (i.n.i.d.). The heterogeneity of the distributions is attributed to the difference between truncation intervals $[u_i, v_i]$'s.

In developing the asymptotic theory, we suggest applying the Lindeberg-Feller CLT or the Lyapunov CLT that deal with the case of i.n.i.d. data. The CLT for i.n.i.d. data is not only applicable to the problem of double-truncation, but also the problems of linear regression (p. 21 of van der Vaart 1998; p. 104 of Lehmann and Romano 2005), stratified sampling (Lehmann 2004), and meta-analysis with differing study variances (Shih et al. 2019). The following theorem is stated whose proof is referred to Emura et al. (2017).

Theorem 2 Let $\boldsymbol{\eta}^0 = (\eta_1^0, \eta_2^0, \ldots, \eta_k^0)^{\mathrm{T}} \in \Theta$ be the true parameter point. Under some regularity conditions stated in Emura et al. (2017),

(a) *Existence and consistency: There exists a solution $\hat{\boldsymbol{\eta}}$ to Eq. (2.2) with probability tending to one, such that $\hat{\boldsymbol{\eta}} \overset{P}{\to} \boldsymbol{\eta}^0$ as $n \to \infty$.*

(b) *Consistency of the observed information matrix: There exists a $k \times k$ positive definite matrix $J(\boldsymbol{\eta})$ such that $-\frac{1}{n} \frac{\partial^2}{\partial \boldsymbol{\eta} \partial \boldsymbol{\eta}^{\mathrm{T}}} \ell(\boldsymbol{\eta})\big|_{\boldsymbol{\eta}=\boldsymbol{\eta}^0} \overset{P}{\to} J(\boldsymbol{\eta}^0)$.*

(c) *Asymptotic normality: $\sqrt{n}(\hat{\boldsymbol{\eta}} - \boldsymbol{\eta}^0) \overset{d}{\to} N_k(\boldsymbol{0}, J^{-1}(\boldsymbol{\eta}^0))$ as $n \to \infty$.*

By Theorem 2(a, b), we have an approximation

$$J(\boldsymbol{\eta}^0) \approx -\frac{1}{n} \frac{\partial^2}{\partial \boldsymbol{\eta} \partial \boldsymbol{\eta}^{\mathrm{T}}} \ell(\boldsymbol{\eta})\bigg|_{\boldsymbol{\eta}=\hat{\boldsymbol{\eta}}}.$$

This and Theorem 2(c) give the normal approximation

$$\hat{\boldsymbol{\eta}} \sim N_k \left(\boldsymbol{\eta}^0, \left\{ -\frac{\partial^2}{\partial \boldsymbol{\eta} \partial \boldsymbol{\eta}^{\mathrm{T}}} \ell(\boldsymbol{\eta}) \bigg|_{\boldsymbol{\eta}=\hat{\boldsymbol{\eta}}} \right\}^{-1} \right).$$

Consequently, the SE for estimating η_j is

$$SE(\hat{\eta}_j) = \sqrt{\left[\left\{ -\frac{\partial^2}{\partial \boldsymbol{\eta} \partial \boldsymbol{\eta}^{\mathrm{T}}} \ell(\boldsymbol{\eta}) \bigg|_{\boldsymbol{\eta}=\hat{\boldsymbol{\eta}}} \right\}^{-1} \right]_{jj}}, \quad j \in \{1, 2, \ldots, k\},$$

and the $(1 - \alpha)100\%$CI for η_j is

$$[\hat{\eta}_j - Z_{\alpha/2} \cdot SE(\hat{\eta}_j), \, \hat{\eta}_j + Z_{\alpha/2} \cdot SE(\hat{\eta}_j)], \quad j \in \{1, 2, \ldots, k\},$$

where Z_p is the pth upper quantile for $N(0, 1)$.

The SE of estimating the survival function is

$$SE\{S_{\hat{\boldsymbol{\eta}}}(y)\} = \sqrt{\left\{ \frac{\partial}{\partial \boldsymbol{\eta}} S_{\boldsymbol{\eta}}(y) \right\}^{\mathrm{T}} \cdot \left\{ -\frac{\partial^2}{\partial \boldsymbol{\eta} \partial \boldsymbol{\eta}^{\mathrm{T}}} \ell(\boldsymbol{\eta}) \right\}^{-1} \cdot \frac{\partial}{\partial \boldsymbol{\eta}} S_{\boldsymbol{\eta}}(y) \bigg|_{\boldsymbol{\eta}=\hat{\boldsymbol{\eta}}}},$$

where

$$\frac{\partial}{\partial \boldsymbol{\eta}} S_{\boldsymbol{\eta}}(y) = \int_{y \in y, t > y} \begin{bmatrix} t - E^1(\boldsymbol{\eta})/E^0(\boldsymbol{\eta}) \\ \vdots \\ t^k - E^k(\boldsymbol{\eta})/E^0(\boldsymbol{\eta}) \end{bmatrix} \cdot f_{\boldsymbol{\eta}}(t) dt.$$

The $(1 - \alpha)100\%$ pointwise CI for the survival function $S_{\boldsymbol{\eta}}(y)$ is

$$\left[S_{\hat{\boldsymbol{\eta}}}(y) - Z_{\alpha/2} \cdot SE\{S_{\hat{\boldsymbol{\eta}}}(y)\}, \, S_{\hat{\boldsymbol{\eta}}}(y) + Z_{\alpha/2} \cdot SE\{S_{\hat{\boldsymbol{\eta}}}(y)\} \right].$$

Example: One-parameter model with $\eta \in \mathbb{R}$
Recall that the survival function is

$$S_{\eta}(y) = \frac{\exp(\eta \tau_2) - \exp(\eta y)}{\exp(\eta \tau_2) - \exp(\eta \tau_1)}, \quad \tau_1 < y < \tau_2.$$

The derivative is

$$\frac{d}{d\eta}S_\eta(y) = \frac{\tau_2 \exp(\eta\tau_2) - y\exp(\eta y)}{\exp(\eta\tau_2) - \exp(\eta\tau_1)} - S_\eta(y)\left\{\frac{\tau_2 \exp(\eta\tau_2) - \tau_1 \exp(\eta y)}{\exp(\eta\tau_2) - \exp(\eta\tau_1)}\right\}.$$

Accordingly, the SE is computed as

$$SE\{S_{\hat{\eta}}(y)\} = \sqrt{\left.\left\{\frac{d}{d\eta}S_\eta(y)\right\}^2 / -\frac{\partial^2}{\partial\eta^2}\ell(\eta)\right|_{\eta=\hat{\eta}}}.$$

The 95%CI for η is

$$[\hat{\eta} - Z_{\alpha/2} \cdot SE(\hat{\eta}), \hat{\eta} + Z_{\alpha/2} \cdot SE(\hat{\eta})].$$

Appendix C includes some R codes for computing the SE and 95%CI.

2.6 An R Package "double.truncation"

We developed the *double.truncation* R package (Emura et al. 2019) that implements various statistical methods for analyzing doubly truncated data. For instance, the package can compute the MLE under various models, where the MLE is obtained by the NR algorithm as stated previously.

Recall that doubly truncated data are expressed as $\{(u_i, y_i, v_i); u_i \le y_i \le v_i, i = 1, 2, \ldots, n\}$. In *double.truncation*, we use the following styles for inputs:

- u.trunc: a vector $(u_1, u_2, \ldots, u_n)$,
- y.trunc: a vector $(y_1, y_2, \ldots, y_n)$,
- v.trunc: a vector $(v_1, v_2, \ldots, v_n)$.

For instance, one can apply *PMLE.SEF3.negative()* to compute the MLE under the cubic model with $\eta_3 < 0$. Below are the outputs of running some simple R codes:

```
library(double.truncation)

u.trunc=c(0,2,5,0)
y.trunc=c(2,5,8,1)
v.trunc=c(3,8,9,7)
PMLE.SEF3.negative(u.trunc,y.trunc,v.trunc, epsilon = 1e-05)
```

The output is shown below

```
$eta
eta1            eta2           eta3
-4.20679283   0.74246155   -0.03959054


$SE
eta1            eta2           eta3
3.37681241    0.76588758    0.05194328


$convergence
logL           DF             AIC            No.of.iterations
-4.152361     3.000000      14.304721     5.000000


$Score
[1] -6.878054e-12 -4.314415e-11 -2.282832e-10


$Hessian
            [,1]            [,2]            [,3]
[1,]   -8.178417      -77.04768      -626.0269
[2,]   -77.047676    -788.36366    -6806.7246
[3,]   -626.026896  -6806.72460   -61509.7506
```

The output above shows the MLE, SE, log-likelihood, degrees of freedom, AIC, and the number of iterations. The log-likelihood, score vector and Hessian matrix are computed at the converged value of the NR algorithm, namely,

$$\log L = \ell(\hat{\eta}), \quad \$Score = \left.\frac{\partial}{\partial \eta}\ell(\eta)\right|_{\eta=\hat{\eta}}, \quad \$Hessian = \left.\frac{\partial^2}{\partial \eta \partial \eta^T}\ell(\eta)\right|_{\eta=\hat{\eta}}.$$

The AIC is defined as

$$\text{AIC} = -2\ell(\hat{\eta}) + 2k.$$

If the values of "$Score=" is not close enough to zero, one may decrease the number in "epsilon $= 1e-05$" that is related to the convergence criterion $\varepsilon > 0$ in the NR algorithm. While a smaller number $\varepsilon > 0$ is desirable, it leads to a larger number of iterations to achieve convergence.

2.7 Data Analysis

We analyze the childhood cancer data obtained from Moreira and de Uña-Álvarez (2010). Their data include the ages at onset of childhood cancer (any cancer occurring before age 15) within a recruitment period of 5 years (between 1 January 1999 and 31 December 2003). The data consist of 406 children with $\{(u_i, y_i, v_i) : i = 1, \ldots, 406\}$ subject to $u_i \leq y_i \leq v_i$, where y_i is the age (in days) at diagnosis, u_i is the age at the start of the recruitment (1 January 1999), and $v_i = u_i + 1825$ is the age at the end of the recruitment (31 December 2003). See Moreira and de Uña-Álvarez (2010) and Chap. 1 for more details about the data.

We set the lower bound $\tau_1 = \min_i(y_i) = 6$ (days) and the upper bound $\tau_2 = \max_i(y_i) = 5474$ (days). Hence, all the observed onset ages belong to the interval $[\tau_1, \tau_2] = [6, 5474]$. Note that this interval almost agrees with to the definition of childhood cancer, any cancer occurring between birth (0 days) and 15 years of age (5475 days).

We fitted the childhood cancer data to seven different models from the SEF as listed in Table 2.2. We applied the NR algorithm of Sect. 2.4 with the convergence criterion $\varepsilon = 0.00001$ for all the considered models, which can be performed through the R package *double.truncation*. We provide our R codes for the data analysis in Appendix C.

We selected a suitable model among the seven models in terms of $\text{AIC} = -2\ell(\hat{\boldsymbol{\eta}}) + 2k$. The chosen model was the one with the minimum AIC value. Table 2.2 shows that the best AIC is attained by the one-parameter model with $\eta \in \mathbb{R}$. Hence, we chose this model for subsequent analyses.

Based on the chosen model, the survival function was estimated by

Table 2.2 Fitted values for the seven different models using the childhood cancer data

Model	$\hat{\eta}_1$	$\hat{\eta}_2$	$\hat{\eta}_3$	$\ell(\hat{\boldsymbol{\eta}})$	k	AIC
1-parameter model ($\eta_1 > 0$)	8.74×10^{-5}	–	–	-3013.6	1	6029.2
1-parameter model ($\eta_1 < 0$)	-3.85×10^{-4}	–	–	-2999.6	1	6001.1
1-parameter model ($\eta_1 \in \mathbb{R}$)	-1.92×10^{-4}	–	–	-2970.4	1	5942.9
2-parameter model ($\eta_2 < 0$)	7.71×10^{-4}	-1.87×10^{-7}	–	-3027.6	2	6059.2
Cubic model ($\eta_3 > 0$)	1.52×10^{-3}	-7.62×10^{-7}	8.92×10^{-11}	-2994.2	3	5994.4
Cubic model ($\eta_3 < 0$)	-7.90×10^{-4}	3.38×10^{-7}	-4.87×10^{-11}	-2991.6	3	5989.2
Cubic model ($\eta_3 \in \mathbb{R}$)	-5.55×10^{-5}	-1.22×10^{-7}	1.94×10^{-11}	-2969.7	3	5945.3

Note $\text{AIC} = -2\ell(\hat{\boldsymbol{\eta}}) + 2k$ (smaller AIC corresponds to better fit)

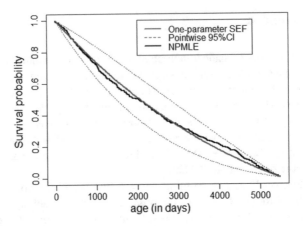

Fig. 2.4 The estimated survival functions obtained from the childhood cancer data. The pointwise 95% CI (for the one-parameter model) is denoted by dotted lines

$$S_{\hat{\eta}}(y) = \frac{\exp(\hat{\eta}\tau_2) - \exp(\hat{\eta}y)}{\exp(\hat{\eta}\tau_2) - \exp(\hat{\eta}\tau_1)}, \quad \tau_1 < y < \tau_2.$$

where $\hat{\eta} = -1.92 \times 10^{-4}$, $\tau_1 = 6$, and $\tau_2 = 5474$. Figure 2.4 depicts the estimated survival function $S_{\hat{\eta}}(y)$ with its 95% pointwise CI. We applied the formulas of Sect. 2.5 to compute the CI.

We compared $S_{\hat{\eta}}(y)$ with the survival function estimated by the NPMLE (see Chap. 3 for the definition). Figure 2.4 shows a similarity of the two estimators of the survival function. This confirms that the one-parameter model with $\eta \in \mathbb{R}$ provides a good fit to the data.

The choice of $\tau_1 = 6$, and $\tau_2 = 5474$ can be changed to $\tau_1 = 0$, and $\tau_2 = 5475$, a period between birth (0 days) and 15 years of age (5475 days). The results of the data analysis essentially stay the same after this change. Readers may refer to Emura et al. (2015) who examined goodness-of-fit for some models based on this period.

2.8 Additional Remarks

In this chapter, what we consider is the conditional likelihood approach, which may be different from the full likelihood approach (see Chaps. 1 and 4). Hence, it would be of great interest to discuss the efficiency and robustness of the MLE. The conditional likelihood approach has the advantage of being free from the distributional assumptions for the truncation limits. On the other hand, it is often natural to utilize the distributional assumptions of the truncation limits into estimation, as in Dörre (2017) and Chap. 3. In particular, the left-truncation limit u_i^* can be regarded a realization from a uniform distribution, and the right-truncation limit is $v_i^* = u_i^* + d_0$, where $d_0 > 0$ is a constant, as in the childhood cancer data. A related paper is de

Uña-Álvarez (2004) who constructed a moment-based estimator that is more efficient than the NPMLE when u_i^* follows a uniform distribution and $v_i^* = u_i^* + d_0$ is a right-censoring limit (instead of right-truncation limit).

Many models in the SEF provide a simple expression for the mode of the density (Sect. 2.2). Hence, one can easily estimate the mode by substituting the MLE to the expression. The SE and CI can also be computed by applying the asymptotic theory and the delta method. For three or more parameters, the delta method may be difficult to apply. In this case, there are several options including a simple bootstrap method of Moreira and de Uña-Álvarez (2010), a parametric bootstrap method, and a more elaborate bootstrap designed for estimating the mode (Mazucheli et al. 2005).

In the SEF, the log-density is approximated by polynomial basis functions. Other basis functions may be employed in a similar fashion, such as spline basis functions. General methodologies are available for approximating the log-density or log-hazard function (O'Sullivan 1998). An alternative is to apply the cubic M-spline basis functions whose R functions are available in the *joint.Cox* package (Emura 2019). For these basis functions, one may directly approximate the density or hazard function without taking "log" since the integral of density or hazard function is explicitly written by I-spline basis functions (Ramsay 1988).

References

Castillo JD (1994) The singly truncated normal distribution: a non-steep exponential family. Ann Inst Stat Math 46:57–66

de Uña-Álvarez J (2004) Nonparametric estimation under length-biased sampling and type I censoring: a moment based approach. Ann Inst Stat Math 56:667–681

Dörre A (2017) Bayesian estimation of a lifetime distribution under double truncation caused by time-restricted data collection. Stat Pap. https://doi.org/10.1007/s00362-017-0968-7

Efron B, Petrosian R (1999) Nonparametric methods for doubly truncated data. J Am Stat Assoc 94:824–834

Emura T (2019) joint.Cox: joint frailty-copula models for tumour progression and death in meta-analysis, CRAN

Emura T, Konno Y, Michimae H (2015) Statistical inference based on the nonparametric maximum likelihood estimator under double-truncation. Lifetime Data Anal 21(3):397–418

Emura T, Hu YH, Konno Y (2017) Asymptotic inference for maximum likelihood estimators under the special exponential family with double-truncation. Stat Pap 58(3):877–909

Emura T, Hu YH, Huang CY (2019) double.truncation: analysis of doubly-truncated data, CRAN

Emura T, Pan CH (2017) Parametric maximum likelihood inference and goodness-of-fit tests for dependently left-truncated data, a copula-based approach. Stat Pap. https://doi.org/10.1007/s00362-017-0947-z

Everitt BS (2003) Modern medical statistics: a practical guide. Arnold, London, United Kingdom

He Z, Emura T (2019) Likelihood inference under the COM-Poisson cure model for survival data—computational aspects. J Chin Stat Assoc 57:1–42

Hu YH, Emura T (2015) Maximum likelihood estimation for a special exponential family under random double-truncation. Comput Stat 30(4):1199–1229

Huang CY, Tseng YK, Emura T (2019) Likelihood-based analysis of doubly-truncated data under the location-scale and AFT model. Comput Stat (in revision)

Knight K (2000) Mathematical statistics. Chapman and Hall, Boca Raton

Lehmann EL, Casella G (1998) Theory of point estimation. Springer, New York

Lehmann EL (2004) Elements of large-sample theory. Springer, New York

Lehmann EL, Romano JP (2005) Testing statistical hypotheses. Springer, New York

Mandrekar SJ, Mandrekar JN (2003) Are our data symmetric? Stat Methods Med Res 12:505–513

McLachlan GJ, McGiffin DC (1994) On the role of finite mixture models in survival analysis. Stat Methods Med Res 3(3):211–226

Moreira C, de Uña-Álvarez J (2010) Bootstrapping the NPMLE for doubly truncated data. J Nonparametr Stat 22:567–583

Matsui S, Sadaike T, Hamada C, Fukushima M (2005) Creutzfeldt-Jakob disease and cadaveric dura mater grafts in Japan: an updated analysis of incubation time. Neuroepidemiology 24:22–25

Mazucheli J, Barros EAC, Achcar JA (2005) Bootstrap confidence intervals for the mode of the hazard function. Comput Methods Programs Biomed 79(1):39–47

O'Sullivan F (1998) Fast computation of fully automated log-density and log-hazard estimation. SIAM J Sci Stat Comput 9:363–379

Ramsay J (1988) Monotone regression spline in action. Stat Sci 3:425–461

Robertson HT, Allison DB (2012) A novel generalized normal distribution for human longevity and other negatively skewed data. PLoS ONE 7:e37025

Shih JH, Konno Y, Chang YT, Emura T (2019) Estimation of a common mean vector in bivariate meta-analysis under the FGM copula. Statistics. https://doi.org/10.1080/02331888.2019.1581782

Shih JH, Emura T (2018) Likelihood-based inference for bivariate latent failure time models with competing risks under the generalized FGM copula. Comput Stat 33(3):1223–1293

Van der Vaart AW (1998) Asymptotic statistics. Cambridge University Press, Cambridge

Chapter 3
Bayesian Inference for Doubly Truncated Data

Abstract Doubly truncated lifetimes can arise under time-restricted availability of observational data. In this case, incorporating information on the birth process of units (i.e. the process which describes the emergence of units in the latent population), whose behaviour might change throughout time, is relevant for statistical inference. In this chapter, a Bayesian approach to double-truncation is developed which allows for piecewise constant process intensities. It is described in detail how a valid likelihood function can be developed for this framework. In addition, estimation of the model is explained with numerical suggestions for efficient implementation. The validity of fitted models is assessed via posterior predictive checks. Finally, the method is applied to the dataset of German insolvent companies in order to estimate the latent lifetime distribution and birth process of companies.

Keywords Bayesian inference · Double-truncation · Likelihood construction · Random sample size · Observational data

3.1 Introduction

In this chapter, we explore a Bayesian view of the problem of double-truncation. The method presented here was originally motivated by a type of observational survival data which is caused by restricted data collection and can be frequently found in practice. In this framework, units of the population of interest are sampled if and only if their death event occurs during the data collection period, which is defined on a calendar time axis. Since units may emerge randomly over time according to a *birth* process, there is no common initial point of the individual lifetimes and thus random truncation occurs. As this birth process is often unknown, the Bayesian approach is set up to adequately deal with this uncertainty.

Figure 3.1 illustrates the data collection scheme as a Lexis diagram where the horizontal axis depicts the calendar time, through which units emerge (*birth*). Depending on the time of their *death*, they may be sampled during the time span (t^L, t^R). This circumstance may typically occur in non-experimental studies such as when registry data are used (see Kalbfleisch and Lawless (1989) for the AIDS dataset, Scheike

© The Author(s), under exclusive license to Springer Nature Singapore Pte Ltd. 2019   41
A. Dörre and T. Emura, *Analysis of Doubly Truncated Data*, JSS Research
Series in Statistics, https://doi.org/10.1007/978-981-13-6241-5_3

Fig. 3.1 Lexis diagram of the data collection scheme. Units are born at random times and sampled if their death occurs during the data collection period (depicted in gray)

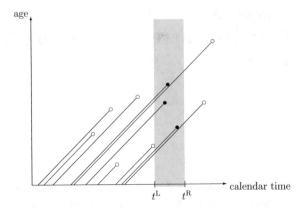

and Keiding (2006) for a study on time-to-pregnancy, West (1996) and Lawless and Kalbfleisch (1992) for related economic contexts). Note however that the presented method can also be applied to modelling controlled experimental data. Depending on the context, the interpretation of the 'birth' process may be different. For instance, for the luminosity data in Efron and Petrosian (1999), the horizontal axis depicts the redshift of stars and thus 'birth' corresponds to the distribution of stars with respect to the redshift seen from earth. Nevertheless, we maintain the notions of *birth*, *lifetime* and *death* throughout this chapter for instructive purposes.

Bayesian inference has been studied in similar selection models (see, for instance, Bayarri and DeGroot (1987), West (1994) and Lee and Berger (2001)) with varying focus. The early contributions of (Sanathanan 1972, 1977) considered truncation in a broad framework and are a fundamental basis of the modelling ideas presented here. Other recent research that inspired the method presented here include Emura and Konno (2012), Emura et al. (2017), Hu and Emura (2015) and Shen (2017).

3.2 Bayesian Inference

We give a brief sketch of the fundamentals of Bayesian inference relevant to the presented method, which may be skipped by readers who are familiar with the subject.

In the framework of Bayesian statistics and Bayesian modelling, uncertainty is generally represented by probability distributions. These distributions can be thought of as the knowledge about model parameters before and after observing data. Since the parameters of the lifetime distribution and the birth process are unknown, we impose distributions on the respective parameter spaces. Subsequently, we are interested in updating the—usually vague—knowledge using the observed data to get another probability distribution on the parameters. We call the former distribution prior (as it is chosen before data are observed) and the latter one posterior distribution. Any inferential aspect concerning the parameters is derived from the posterior distribution. In fact, a somewhat immediate estimate of the parameters is already given by the posterior distribution itself.

In addition to introducing a probabilistic model to express the uncertainty about the parameters, the Bayesian approach offers a mathematically sound way of describing how the data affect the information one has about the parameters. Let γ denote some generic vector-valued parameter and D denote the data. Two fundamental ingredients are required: the prior density $\pi(\cdot)$ defined on the parameter space and the likelihood function $\ell(\cdot|D)$, which is defined as the density of the data given a set of parameters. The primary result of the Bayesian approach is the posterior density $\pi(\cdot|D)$, which is formally defined as the density of the parameters given the data.

The posterior density is acquired by applying Bayes' rule on the parameters γ given the data. This leads to

$$\pi(\gamma|D) = \frac{\ell(\gamma|D)\pi(\gamma)}{\int \ell(\gamma|D)\pi(\gamma)d\gamma}. \tag{3.1}$$

Note that the denominator in Eq. (3.1) represents the normalizing constant of the posterior density, which ensures that the posterior density integrates to 1. Moreover, as γ is integrated out in the denominator in Eq. (3.1), it does not affect the shape of the posterior density. In other words, since $\int \pi(\gamma|D)d\gamma$ must equal 1 for given data D, the complete posterior density can be recovered from just considering its shape (see Eq. (3.2) below).

Once the posterior distribution is obtained, inference on any aspect of the involved parameters can be conducted. Usually, the posterior mean (i.e. the mean of the posterior distribution) is used as a basic point estimate, while the posterior variance serves as an indication of the uncertainty contained in the posterior distribution. It is worth noting that the posterior variance asymptotically coincides with the frequentist notion of the variance of the estimator, under mild regularity conditions.

By choosing the likelihood model and a prior distribution, we implicitly define a joint probabilistic model of (γ, D). The marginal density of the data is given as $f(D) = \int \ell(\gamma|D)\pi(\gamma)d\gamma$ and so the posterior density can be briefly written as

$$\pi(\gamma|D) = \frac{\ell(\gamma|D)\pi(\gamma)}{f(D)}.$$

Furthermore, the term $f(D)$ evidently does not depend on γ (as it is the marginal density of the data) and thus, when neglecting all terms in $\pi(\gamma|D)$ that are constant with respect to γ, we can write

$$\pi(\gamma|D) \propto \ell(\gamma|D)\pi(\gamma). \tag{3.2}$$

The posterior distribution is fully characterized by the right-hand side of Eq. (3.2), as the normalizing constant can be reconstructed via integrating this proportional term, i.e. $C = \int \ell(\gamma|D)\pi(\gamma)d\gamma$.

This technical simplification will become useful later during estimation, since the normalizing constant is difficult to determine in many situations, but is not required for obtaining the posterior mean and the posterior variance.

In some special cases, it is possible to find a class of prior distributions such that the posterior distribution is in the same distribution class. In this case, the prior distribution is called conjugate for the likelihood function. For conjugate priors, determining the posterior distribution, therefore, reduces to adequately updating the prior parameters. As an example, consider a sample of size n from the exponential distribution, i.e.

$$f(y_1, \ldots, y_n|\theta) = \theta^n e^{-\theta \sum_{i=1}^n y_i}, \qquad y > 0$$

for some unknown θ. If we assume that the prior distribution of θ is a Gamma distribution with parameters α_0 and β_0, then

$$\pi(\theta) = \frac{\beta_0^{\alpha_0}}{\Gamma(\alpha_0)} \cdot \theta^{\alpha_0-1} e^{-\beta_0\theta}, \qquad \theta > 0,$$

and the kernel, i.e. the essential algebraic part of the density neglecting normalizing terms, of the posterior distribution is given as

$$\pi(\theta|y_1, \ldots, y_n) \propto \theta^n e^{-\theta \sum_{i=1}^n y_i} \cdot \frac{\beta_0^{\alpha_0}}{\Gamma(\alpha_0)} \cdot \theta^{\alpha_0-1} e^{-\beta_0\theta}$$

$$\propto \theta^n e^{-\theta \sum_{i=1}^n y_i} \cdot \theta^{\alpha_0-1} e^{-\beta_0\theta}$$

$$= \theta^{\alpha_0+n-1} e^{-\theta(\beta_0 + \sum_{i=1}^n y_i)},$$

which is again the kernel of a Gamma distribution with parameters $\alpha_n = \alpha_0 + n$ and $\beta_n = \beta_0 + \sum y_i$. Simulating from a Gamma distribution is straightforward using any statistical software such as R. Therefore, conjugacy directly enables assessing the posterior distribution in this example.

However, in many situations, conjugate priors are either not available or too unpleasant to handle. By using MCMC (Markov Chain Monte Carlo) methods the exact determination of the posterior distribution can be circumvented and instead an approximate sample of any desired size from it is drawn. This is particularly convenient since a posterior sample, broadly speaking, is a discrete pseudo-empirical representation of the posterior distribution and any aspect including its moments, percentiles, etc. can be readily approximated.

The Bayesian methodology proves particularly helpful for the considered model with calendar time structure. This is because the uncertainty about the birth process can be included in the Bayesian model right away. Specifically, based on a parametric representation of the birth process, we obtain two types of parameters—lifetime and birth process parameters—for which we consider the posterior distribution given data. For this to be attainable, we first investigate the truncation mechanism and derive a proper likelihood model.

3.3 A Bayesian Model for Double-Truncation

For any statistical method based on the likelihood principle, establishing an appropriate and manageable likelihood model for the data is a central task. When truncation is considered, the selection phenomenon needs to be reflected in this endeavour, too. As there is no unique way of doing this, several fundamental ideas have emerged in the literature (see Wang (1989)).

For building a likelihood model, we employ a fundamental relation of densities under random sample sizes. Suppose that we consider an infinite sequence of *iid* random variables $z_i, i \in \mathbb{N}$, distributed according to some density $f(\cdot|\boldsymbol{\theta})$, of which we observe a random number of elements $z_1, \ldots, z_n$. Taking into account that n is a random variable, whose distribution may depend on $\boldsymbol{\theta}$ and on an additional parameter λ, the density is given as

$$f(n, z_1, \ldots, z_n | \lambda, \boldsymbol{\theta}) = f(z_1, \ldots, z_n | \lambda, \boldsymbol{\theta}, n) \cdot f(n | \lambda, \boldsymbol{\theta}) = \prod_{i=1}^{n} f(z_i | \boldsymbol{\theta}) \cdot f(n | \lambda, \boldsymbol{\theta}),$$

$$(3.3)$$

where $f(n|\lambda, \boldsymbol{\theta})$ denotes the density function of n. By this equation the joint density of n and $z_1, \ldots, z_n$ is decomposed into two parts, of which the first factor does not involve λ. The parameter λ is chosen below as the intensity $\lambda(\cdot)$ of a Poisson process, which describes the emergence (birth) of units in the population and implicitly governs the behaviour of the random sample size.

In the following, we generally denote the random birth and lifetime of a unit in the latent population by b^* and y^*, and the corresponding random values of a sample unit are denoted by b and y. It is generally assumed that b^* and y^* are independent. We denote the density and distribution function of y^* as $f(\cdot|\boldsymbol{\theta})$ and $F(\cdot|\boldsymbol{\theta})$, respectively; the random births b^* are distributed according to $g(\cdot|\lambda(\cdot))$ and $G(\cdot|\lambda(\cdot))$.

3.3.1 Birth Process

We generally model the emergence of new units during calendar time as a Poisson process on an overall birth interval $[s, t]$, which precedes the observation interval (t^L, t^R):

$$N(A)|\lambda(\cdot) \sim \text{Poi}\left(\int_A \lambda(b)db\right), \qquad A \subseteq [s, t]$$

This means that for any given subset A of the birth interval $[s, t]$, we suppose that the number of latent units in A, denoted by $N(A)$, is Poisson distributed with parameter $\Lambda(A) = \int_A \lambda(b)db$. In addition, for $N(\cdot)$ being a proper Poisson process on $[s, t]$, we implicitly require that

- units are born independent of each other, i.e. for disjoint sets $A_1, \ldots, A_m, m \in \mathbb{N}$, the random variables $N(A_1), \ldots, N(A_m)$, are independent (in particular, one birth does not affect the process intensity before or after it; thus implying a notion of memorylessness)
- units are born separately, i.e. never at the same time
- the number of units born before some point in time x is Poisson distributed, i.e.

$$N([s, x]) \sim \text{Poi} \left(\int_s^x \lambda(b)db \right)$$

By modelling the population size as a random variable, we avoid considering the random sample size conditional on the discrete variable N, which would be technically less appealing. In this birth process model, the probability density function of latent births is generally implied as

$$g(b|\lambda(\cdot)) = \frac{\lambda(b)}{\int_{[s,t]} \lambda(b)db} = \lambda(b)/\Lambda, \qquad b \in [s, t]. \tag{3.4}$$

It is interesting to note that this density function is invariant with respect to scaling of the birth intensity. In particular, when considering the normalized version $\widetilde{\lambda}$ of the birth intensity, i.e. $\widetilde{\lambda}(b) = \lambda(b)/\Lambda$, we obtain the same distribution of latent births:

$$g(b|\widetilde{\lambda}(\cdot)) = g(b|\lambda(\cdot)). \tag{3.5}$$

3.3.2 Selection Probability

It is a key assumption in our investigation that the sample size n is a random variable. Furthermore, as we establish a joint model for the births and lifetimes (b, y), there is a common probability

$$p(\lambda(\cdot), \boldsymbol{\theta}) = \text{P}(t^L \leq b^* + y^* \leq t^R | \lambda(\cdot), \boldsymbol{\theta}) \tag{3.6}$$

for all units in the population to be selected into the observed sample. It is important to note that this *selection probability* depends simultaneously on the birth distribution and the lifetime distribution, as the selection criterion evidently depends on both variables b^* and y^*. Therefore, both parts, birth and lifetime distribution, need to be considered (at least to some extent) in order to estimate the lifetime distribution. Depending on the particular choice of the intensity function $\lambda(\cdot)$ and the lifetime parameters $\boldsymbol{\theta}$, different selection probabilities and lifetime densities result. However, the general relations Eqs. (3.3) and (3.6) are always valid and thus not affected. One slightly surprising fact is that the birth process need not necessarily be fully estimated. In fact, it is impossible to find a consistent estimator of the entire birth process intensity function.

Suppose that the population size N is Poisson distributed with parameter Λ and n is the sample size resulting from selecting units from the population with common selection probability p. Then n is conditionally binomially distributed given N and p; in short: $N|\Lambda \sim \text{Poi}(\Lambda)$ and $n|N, p \sim \text{Bin}(N, p)$. We are interested in deriving the unconditional distribution of n, as N is generally unknown.

Proposition 3.1 *Suppose that $N|\Lambda \sim \text{Poi}(\Lambda)$ and $n|N, p \sim \text{Bin}(N, p)$. Then n is (unconditionally) Poisson distributed as $n|\Lambda, p \sim \text{Poi}(p \cdot \Lambda)$, i.e.*

$$P(n = k|\Lambda, p) = \frac{(\Lambda p)^k}{k!} e^{-\Lambda p} \quad \forall k \in \mathbb{N}_0.$$

Proof In order to show that the sample size n is Poisson distributed with parameter $p\Lambda$, we directly calculate the probability density function of n. For this, let $k \in \mathbb{N}_0$.

For n to be equal to k, two requirements need to be fulfilled: (1) the underlying random population size N needs to be some integer $\geq k$ and (2) the sample size represents k successful binomial draws from N with probability p. Therefore,

$$
\begin{aligned}
P(n = k|\Lambda, p) &= \sum_{N'=k}^{\infty} P(n = k|p, N = N') \cdot P(N = N'|\Lambda) \\
&= \sum_{N'=k}^{\infty} \binom{N'}{k} p^k (1 - p)^{N'-k} \cdot \frac{\Lambda^{N'}}{N'!} e^{-\Lambda} \\
&= \frac{(p\Lambda)^k}{k!} \cdot \sum_{N'=k}^{\infty} \frac{1}{(N' - k)!} (1 - p)^{N'-k} \cdot \Lambda^{N'-k} e^{-\Lambda} \\
&= \frac{(p\Lambda)^k}{k!} \cdot \sum_{N'=0}^{\infty} \frac{((1 - p)\Lambda)^{N'}}{N'!} e^{-\Lambda} \\
&= \frac{(\Lambda p)^k}{k!} \cdot e^{\Lambda(1-p)} \cdot e^{-\Lambda} \\
&= \frac{(\Lambda p)^k}{k!} e^{-\Lambda p}.
\end{aligned}
$$

Since $k \in \mathbb{N}_0$ is arbitrary, it is proven that

$$P(n = k|\Lambda, p) = \frac{(\Lambda p)^k}{k!} e^{-\Lambda p} \quad \forall k \in \mathbb{N}_0,$$

which means that n is Poisson distributed with parameter Λp. $\qquad\square$

Fig. 3.2 Depiction of the
selection mechanism. Lower
panel shows the latent birth
process which is assumed to
be a Poisson process. The
upper panel shows the
observable region of pairs
(b, y) delimited by t^L and t^R

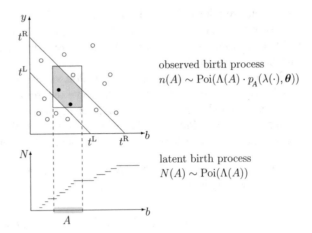

observed birth process
$n(A) \sim \text{Poi}(\Lambda(A) \cdot p_A(\lambda(\cdot), \boldsymbol{\theta}))$

latent birth process
$N(A) \sim \text{Poi}(\Lambda(A))$

Figure 3.2 illustrates the birth process and selection mechanism. As described, units in the population are born according to a Poisson process and selected into the sample if $t^L \leq b^* + y^* \leq t^R$. When a certain subinterval A of the overall birth interval is considered, the observable region of pairs (b, y) constitutes a polygonal shape as displayed in Fig. 3.2. Note that the observed random subsample size with respect to the set A depends on the selection probability $p_A(\lambda(\cdot), \theta)$, which is defined condtional on $b^* \in A$. When $A = [s, t]$, the function p_A equates the selection probability defined above. Proposition 3.1 shows that the sample size n and subinterval sample sizes $n(A)$ are Poisson distributed.

3.3.3 Homogeneous and Inhomogeneous Birth Processes

The simplest model for a birth process consists in choosing $\lambda(\cdot)$ to be constant, by which a homogeneous birth process is defined. In this case, the cumulative birth intensity is proportional to the birth interval, i.e. $\Lambda([s, t]) = \lambda(t - s)$ and the selection probability solely depends on $\boldsymbol{\theta}$. Therefore, when $\lambda(\cdot)$ is constant, $n|\lambda, \boldsymbol{\theta} \sim \text{Poi}(\lambda(t - s)p(\boldsymbol{\theta}))$.

In many practical situations, assuming a homogeneous birth process is too strict, however. As a natural generalization, one might consider piecewise constant birth intensities instead. In particular, we may divide the overall birth interval $[s, t]$ into a finite number of disjoint intervals, which we call birth periods, and equip these with constant intensities λ_k each, while the distribution parameter $\boldsymbol{\theta}$ is assumed to be stationary through calendar time.

By partitioning the birth interval into separate periods $[s_1, t_1), \ldots, [s_m, t_m)$, we consequently obtain disjoint subsamples corresponding to each chosen birth period. The number of observed units within each period is denoted by n_k and it holds that

$$n_k|\lambda_k, \boldsymbol{\theta} \sim \text{Poi}(\lambda_k(t_k - s_k)p_k(\boldsymbol{\theta})), \tag{3.7}$$

where $p_k(\boldsymbol{\theta})$ is defined as the period-specific selection probability.

3.3.4   Density of Observed Lifetimes

In order to fully set up the likelihood function, besides considering the birth process and selection probability we need to establish the density function of the observed lifetimes after truncation. The density of an observed lifetime is mathematically derived as the conditional density of y^* given that the selection criterion is fulfilled for given parameters of the birth process and the latent lifetime distribution. For this, we first suppose that the birth process is a homogeneous Poisson process on the entire birth interval $[s, t]$. As a consequence, the births are uniformly distributed on $[s, t]$. In this case, the following Lemma yields the desired lifetime density.

Lemma 3.1 *Let b^* be uniformly distributed on $[s, t]$. The density function of a single observed lifetime y is then given by*

$$f(y|\theta, t^L \le b^* + y^* \le t^R) = \frac{f(y|\theta)}{p(\theta)} \cdot \frac{t_*^R(y) - t_*^L(y)}{t - s}, \qquad y \in [t^L - t, t^R - s]$$

(3.8)

where

$$t_*^L(y) := \min(\max(t^L - y, s), t) \quad and \quad t_*^R(y) := \min(\max(t^R - y, s), t),$$

and the selection probability $p(\lambda(\cdot), \theta) \equiv p(\theta)$ only depends on θ.

Proof By Bayes' theorem, it holds that

$$
\begin{aligned}
f(y|t^L \le b^* + y^* \le t^R, \theta) &= \frac{f(y, t^L \le b^* + y^* \le t^R|\theta)}{P(t^L \le b^* + y^* \le t^R|\theta)} \\
&= \frac{f(y, t^L \le b^* + y^* \le t^R|\theta)}{p(\lambda(\cdot), \theta)}.
\end{aligned}
$$

Note that b^* being uniformly distributed on $[s, t]$ is equivalent to $\lambda(\cdot) \equiv \lambda$ being constant. This implies $g(b|\lambda(\cdot)) = \frac{\lambda}{\lambda \cdot (t-s)} = \frac{1}{t-s}$ (see Eq. (3.4)). As a consequence, and since b^* and y^* are assumed to be independent,

$$p(\lambda, \theta) = P(t^L \le b^* + y^* \le t^R|\theta) \tag{3.9}$$

$$= \int_{[s,t]} \int_0^\infty f(y^*|\theta) g(b^*|\lambda) \cdot I(t^L \le b^* + y^* \le t^R)\, dy^* db^*$$

$$= \frac{1}{t-s} \int_{[s,t]} \int_0^\infty f(y^*|\theta) \cdot I(t^L \le b^* + y^* \le t^R)\, dy^* db^*,$$

which does not depend on λ. Furthermore, we obtain for the joint density

$$f(y, t^L \leq b^* + y^* \leq t^R | \boldsymbol{\theta}) = \int_s^t f(y|\boldsymbol{\theta}) \frac{1}{t-s} I(t^L \leq b^* + y \leq t^R) \, db^*$$

$$= f(y|\boldsymbol{\theta}) \frac{1}{t-s} \int_s^t I(t^L - y \leq b^* \leq t^R - y) \, db^*$$

$$= f(y|\boldsymbol{\theta}) \frac{1}{t-s} \int_{\min(\max(t^L - y, s), t)}^{\min(\max(t^R - y, s), t)} 1 \, db^*$$

$$= f(y|\boldsymbol{\theta}) \frac{1}{t-s} (t_*^R(y) - t_*^L(y)),$$

which proves the assertion.   □

The extension to piecewise homogeneous Poisson processes as mentioned in Sect. 3.3.3, i.e. to m birth periods with constant birth intensities, follows analogously by noting that such processes can be understood as the sum of m independent Poisson processes each having constant birth intensity. In particular, the random period sub-sample sizes (see Eq. (3.7)) are independent Poisson distributed random variables. From Lemma 3.1, we immediately deduce that

$$f(y|\boldsymbol{\theta}, t^L \leq b^* + y^* \leq t^R, b^* \in [s_k, t_k)) \propto \frac{f(y|\boldsymbol{\theta})}{p_k(\boldsymbol{\theta})}, \quad y \in [t^L - t_k, t^R - s_k],$$

is the lifetime density kernel at y for an individual born in $[s_k, t_k)$.

3.3.5 Likelihood Function

Combining Eq. (3.3) and Proposition 3.1 further yields the likelihood function

$$\ell(\lambda_1, ..., \lambda_m, \boldsymbol{\theta} | n_1, ..., n_m, \mathbf{y}) \propto \prod_{i=1}^n \frac{f(y_i|\boldsymbol{\theta})}{p_{k_i}(\boldsymbol{\theta})} \cdot \prod_{k=1}^m \frac{(\lambda_k(t_k - s_k) p_k(\boldsymbol{\theta}))^{n_k}}{n_k!} e^{-\lambda_k(t_k - s_k) p_k(\boldsymbol{\theta})}$$

$$= \prod_{i=1}^n f(y_i|\boldsymbol{\theta}) \cdot \prod_{k=1}^m \frac{(\lambda_k(t_k - s_k))^{n_k}}{n_k!} e^{-\lambda_k(t_k - s_k) p_k(\boldsymbol{\theta})},$$

where k_i is the period in which the ith observed unit is born. Note that the terms involving $p_k(\boldsymbol{\theta})$ get canceled out. By neglecting all terms constant with respect to $\boldsymbol{\theta}$, we see that the data $D = (n_1, ..., n_m, \mathbf{y})$, consisting of the m subsample sizes $n_1, ..., n_m$ and the observed lifetimes $\mathbf{y} = (y_1, ..., y_n)$ possess the likelihood function proportional to

$$\ell(\lambda_1, ..., \lambda_m, \boldsymbol{\theta} | n_1, ..., n_m, \mathbf{y}) \propto \prod_{i=1}^{n} f(y_i | \boldsymbol{\theta}) \prod_{k=1}^{m} \lambda_k^{n_k} e^{-\lambda_k (t_k - s_k) p_k(\boldsymbol{\theta})}.$$

3.3.6 Identifiability

In order to ensure that the proposed likelihood function is appropriate for statistical inference, we consider the identifiability of the involved parameters. Specifically, we want to show that the likelihood model defined above is unique for any given set of parameters $\lambda_1, ..., \lambda_m, \boldsymbol{\theta}$. In other words, we want to rule out the possibility that the distribution of the data D may be the result of different parameter sets, in which case consistent estimation is impossible. On the other hand, note that identifiability in the sense presented here does not guarantee that a consistent estimator exists. More precisely, the intensity function $b \mapsto \lambda(b)$ of the birth process does not possess a consistent estimator—instead we show that its normalized counterpart $\widetilde{\lambda}(b) := \lambda(b) / \int_{[s,t]} \lambda(b) db$ does. We impose the following assumptions:

(A1) The latent births emerge according to a Poisson process N^b with intensity function $\lambda(\cdot)$.
(A2) The latent lifetimes y_i^* are *iid* according to a continuous density $f(\cdot | \boldsymbol{\theta})$ with support $\mathbb{R}_{\geq 0}$.
(A3) The latent births b_i^* and lifetimes y_i^* are independent.
(A4) If $\exists c : f(y | \boldsymbol{\theta}) = c \cdot f(y | \boldsymbol{\theta}') \ \forall y \in [t^L - t, t^R - s]$, then $\boldsymbol{\theta} = \boldsymbol{\theta}'$,

Concerning assumption (A4), it is demanded that if two density functions agree up to a constant on the observable range $[t^L - t, t^R - s]$ of lifetimes, then the respective parameter sets $\boldsymbol{\theta}$ and $\boldsymbol{\theta}'$ need to be the same.

Lemma 3.2 *Under (A1)–(A4), the parameters $\widetilde{\lambda}(\cdot)$ and $\boldsymbol{\theta}$ are identifiable with respect to the density function*

$$\frac{g(\cdot | \lambda(\cdot)) f(\cdot | \boldsymbol{\theta})}{p(\lambda(\cdot), \boldsymbol{\theta})}.$$

Proof The idea of the proof is to show how the densities f and g can be recovered from any given joint distribution of (b, y) conditional on selection. It is argued that f and g are uniquely derived under the given conditions, which is equivalent to identifiability of $\lambda(\cdot)$ and $\boldsymbol{\theta}$. For any (b, y), define

$$\varphi(b, y | \lambda(\cdot), \boldsymbol{\theta}) := \int_s^b \int_0^y \frac{g(\tilde{b} | \lambda(\cdot)) f(\tilde{y} | \boldsymbol{\theta})}{p(\lambda(\cdot), \boldsymbol{\theta})} I(t^L \leq \tilde{b} + \tilde{y} \leq t^R) d\tilde{y} d\tilde{b}$$

as the cumulative distribution function with respect to the selection set $S := \{(b, y) : t^L \leq b + y \leq t^R\}$. Given that g and f are differentiable almost everywhere, the partial derivatives of φ exist and

$$\omega(b, y|\lambda(\cdot), \boldsymbol{\theta}) := \frac{\partial^2 \varphi(b, y|\lambda(\cdot), \boldsymbol{\theta})}{\partial y \partial b} = \frac{g(b|\lambda(\cdot)) f(y|\boldsymbol{\theta})}{p(\lambda(\cdot), \boldsymbol{\theta})} I(t^L \leq b + y \leq t^R)$$

$$(3.10)$$

is the joint density at (b, y) for given $\lambda(\cdot)$ and $\boldsymbol{\theta}$. Analogously, we obtain the conditional density $\omega(y|b, \lambda(\cdot), \boldsymbol{\theta})$ at y given birth time b by calculating

$$\omega(y|b, \lambda(\cdot), \boldsymbol{\theta}) = \frac{\omega(b, y|\lambda(\cdot), \boldsymbol{\theta})}{\omega(b|\lambda(\cdot), \boldsymbol{\theta})} = \frac{g(b|\lambda(\cdot)) f(y|\boldsymbol{\theta})}{p(\lambda(\cdot), \boldsymbol{\theta})} I((b, y) \in S) \cdot \frac{1}{\int_{t^L-b}^{t^R-b} \omega(b, y|\lambda(\cdot), \boldsymbol{\theta}) dy}$$

$$= \frac{f(y|\boldsymbol{\theta})}{F(\mathcal{Y}_b|\boldsymbol{\theta})} I((b, y) \in S),$$

where $\mathcal{Y}_b := \{y : (b, y) \in S\}$ is the observable range of y, given birth b and the last equation follows by plugging in Eq. (3.10). Note that $\omega(y|b, \lambda(\cdot), \boldsymbol{\theta})$ is in fact invariant with respect to $\lambda(\cdot)$. Fix any $y' \in (t^L - t, t^R - s)$ with $f(y'|\boldsymbol{\theta}) > 0$. For any $y \in \mathcal{Y}_b$, we obtain

$$\frac{\omega(y|b, \lambda(\cdot), \boldsymbol{\theta})}{\omega(y'|b, \lambda(\cdot), \boldsymbol{\theta})} = \frac{f(y|\boldsymbol{\theta})}{f(y'|\boldsymbol{\theta})}$$

if $y' \in \mathcal{Y}_b$. Now suppose that an arbitrary $y \in (t^L - t, t^R - s)$ is given. Since $t^R - t^L > 0$, there exists a finite sequence $(b_1, y_1), \ldots, (b_k, y_k)$ such that $y_1 = y'$, $y_k = y$ and

$$y_j \in \mathcal{Y}_{b_{j-1}} \cap \mathcal{Y}_{b_j} \ \forall j = 2, \ldots, k.$$

It holds that

$$\prod_{j=2}^{k} \frac{\omega(y_j|b_j, \lambda(\cdot), \boldsymbol{\theta})}{\omega(y_{j-1}|b_{j-1}, \lambda(\cdot), \boldsymbol{\theta})} = \frac{f(y|\boldsymbol{\theta})}{f(y'|\boldsymbol{\theta})}$$

Thus the density function $f(\cdot|\boldsymbol{\theta})$ can be determined up to a constant given $\lambda(\cdot)$ and $\boldsymbol{\theta}$. Now suppose that $(\lambda(\cdot), \boldsymbol{\theta})$ and $(\lambda'(\cdot), \boldsymbol{\theta}')$ lead to the same joint distribution φ of (b, y). According to the derivations above, there exists a constant $c = f(y|\boldsymbol{\theta})/f(y|\boldsymbol{\theta}')$ such that

$$f(y|\boldsymbol{\theta}') = c \cdot f(y|\boldsymbol{\theta}) \quad \text{a.e. on } (t^L - t, t^R - s).$$

Due to (A4), it follows that $\boldsymbol{\theta}' = \boldsymbol{\theta}$. Furthermore, by the condition that g integrates to 1, it holds that

$$\int_s^t \frac{\omega(b, y_b|\lambda(\cdot), \boldsymbol{\theta})}{f(y_b|\boldsymbol{\theta})} db = \int_s^t \frac{g(b|\lambda(\cdot))}{p(\lambda(\cdot), \boldsymbol{\theta})} db = \frac{1}{p(\lambda(\cdot), \boldsymbol{\theta})},$$

where each $y_b \in \mathcal{Y}_b$, respectively. Finally, since $g(b|\lambda(\cdot))$ is equal to the derivative of

$$\int_s^b g(\tilde{b}|\lambda(\cdot))d\tilde{b} = \int_s^b \frac{\omega(\tilde{b}, y_{\tilde{b}}|\lambda(\cdot), \boldsymbol{\theta})}{f(y_{\tilde{b}}|\boldsymbol{\theta})} p(\lambda(\cdot), \boldsymbol{\theta})d\tilde{b} = p(\lambda(\cdot), \boldsymbol{\theta}) \int_s^b \frac{\omega(\tilde{b}, y_{\tilde{b}}|\lambda(\cdot), \boldsymbol{\theta})}{f(y_{\tilde{b}}|\boldsymbol{\theta})} d\tilde{b},$$

and since g is identifiable on $[s, t]$ in the population, it can be recovered from the joint density ω. As mentioned before,

$$\tilde{\lambda}(b) = g(b|\lambda(\cdot))$$

and thus $\tilde{\lambda}(\cdot)$ is identifiable. $\qquad\square$

3.3.7 Exponential Families as a Special Case

Exponential families cover many typical distributions used in statistics. For this important special case, for which identifiability is usually not an issue, we show that the truncated model allows a representation as an exponential family, too. Furthermore, we demonstrate that the resulting sufficient statistic is of a particularly convenient type.

Example 1 **Gamma distribution**
We consider the Gamma distribution as an example and assume an overall homogeneous birth process yielding a single observed sample size n for the sake of comprehensibility. It is, however, no additional technical burden to extend the exposition to the case of a piecewise homogeneous birth process (see Sect. 3.3.5). The density functions of one and a sample of n latent lifetimes are given as

$$f(y|\alpha, \beta) = \frac{\beta^\alpha}{\Gamma(\alpha)} \cdot y^{\alpha-1} e^{-\beta y}$$

$$f(\mathbf{y}|\alpha, \beta) = \prod_{i=1}^n f(y_i|\alpha, \beta) = \exp\left(n(\alpha \ln \beta - \ln \Gamma(\alpha)) + (\alpha - 1)\sum_{i=1}^n \ln y_i - \beta \sum_{i=1}^n y_i\right),$$

where the sufficient statistic is $\tilde{\mathbf{T}}_n(\mathbf{y}) = (\sum \ln y_i, \sum y_i)$. Subject to truncation, we obtain the density

$$f(n, \mathbf{y}|\lambda, \alpha, \beta) \propto \prod_{i=1}^n f(y_i|\alpha, \beta) \cdot \exp\left(n \ln \lambda - \lambda(t - s)p(\alpha, \beta)\right),$$

where all factors which are constant with respect to the parameters λ, α and β are omitted and $p(\alpha, \beta)$ is the selection probability

$$
\begin{aligned}
p(\alpha, \beta) &= P(t^L \leq b^* + y^* \leq t^R | \alpha, \beta) \\
&= \frac{1}{t - s} \int\limits_{[s,t]} \int\limits_0^\infty f(y^* | \alpha, \beta) \cdot I(t^L \leq b^* + y^* \leq t^R)\, dy^* db^* \\
&= \frac{1}{t - s} \int\limits_{[s,t]} F(t^R - b^* | \alpha, \beta) - F(t^L - b^* | \alpha, \beta)\, db^*
\end{aligned}
$$

as in Eq. (3.9). Altogether we obtain

$$
f(n, \mathbf{y} | \lambda, \alpha, \beta) = C(\lambda, \alpha, \beta) \cdot \exp\{Q(\lambda, \alpha, \beta) \cdot \mathbf{T}(n, \mathbf{y})\}
$$

with the functions

$$
\begin{aligned}
C(\lambda, \alpha, \beta) &= \exp(-\lambda(t - s)p(\alpha, \beta)) \\
Q(\lambda, \alpha, \beta) &= (\ln \lambda + \alpha \ln \beta - \ln \Gamma(\alpha), \alpha - 1, -\beta) \\
\mathbf{T}(n, \mathbf{y}) &= \left(n, \sum \ln y_i, \sum y_i\right) = \left(n, \tilde{\mathbf{T}}_n(\mathbf{y})\right).
\end{aligned}
$$

Therefore, the model maintains the exponential family property after truncation. It is interesting to note that the sufficient statistic after truncation consists of the sample size n and the original sufficient statistic $\tilde{\mathbf{T}}_n(\mathbf{y})$ of the latent model. In the case of the piecewise constant birth intensity, we similarly obtain $(n_1, \ldots, n_m, \tilde{\mathbf{T}}_n(\mathbf{y}))$, which demonstrates that the dimension of the sufficient statistic is proportional to the number of change points in the birth intensity.

3.4 Estimation

Applying the Bayesian framework to our setting, we define a prior density on the parameters $\lambda_1, \ldots, \lambda_m, \boldsymbol{\theta}$, and determine the kernel of the posterior density:

$$
\pi(\lambda_1, \ldots, \lambda_m, \boldsymbol{\theta} | n_1, \ldots, n_m, \mathbf{y}) \propto \ell(\lambda_1, \ldots, \lambda_m, \boldsymbol{\theta} | n_1, \ldots, n_m, \mathbf{y}) \cdot \pi(\lambda_1, \ldots, \lambda_m, \boldsymbol{\theta}).
\tag{3.11}
$$

It can be shown that there is no convenient conjugate prior distribution for this likelihood model, which is mainly due to the truncation mechanism. For instance, if the latent lifetimes are exponentially distributed (as in a previous Example), a Gamma prior for θ is conjugate in the latent model. However, the kernel of the posterior density, which for $m = 1$ is given as

$$\pi(\lambda, \theta | n, \mathbf{y}) \propto \theta^n e^{-\theta \sum_{i=1}^{n} y_i} \lambda^n e^{-\lambda(b-a)p(\theta)} \cdot \pi(\lambda, \theta),$$

does not admit a direct simple choice of prior distributions for neither θ nor λ due to the multiplicative connection of λ and θ in the term $\exp\{-\lambda(b-a)p(\theta)\}$. Therefore, we move to MCMC methods to simulate the posterior distribution.

3.4.1 Metropolis Algorithm

In order to determine the posterior mean, one would ideally exactly determine the posterior distribution (including its distribution class and parameters). Unfortunately, this approach is not possible in the present situation due to the relatively inconvenient shape of the posterior distribution. The standard solution in this case is to use MCMC algorithms, by which an (approximate) sample from the posterior distribution is generated (see Tierney (1994) for a general investigation of MCMC methods for Bayesian models). This algorithm is defined as follows.

0. Set an initial value γ_0 and $t := 0$.
1. Increase t by 1 and draw $\gamma^* \sim q(\cdot | \gamma_{t-1})$.
2. Calculate r as

$$r(\gamma_{t-1}, \gamma^*) = \min\left(\frac{\pi(\gamma^*|D)q(\gamma_{t-1}|\gamma^*)}{\pi(\gamma_{t-1}|D)q(\gamma^*|\gamma_{t-1})}\right)$$

and draw $u \sim U(0, 1)$.
4. If $r < u$, set $\gamma_t = \gamma^*$, else set $\gamma_t = \gamma_{t-1}$.
5. Repeat steps 1–3 until $t = M$.

Using this algorithm for $\gamma = (\lambda_1, \ldots, \lambda_m, \theta)$, we obtain a sequence $(\lambda_1^j, \ldots, \lambda_m^j, \theta^j)$ of any desired length M, whose elements are approximately $\pi(\lambda_1, \ldots, \lambda_m, \theta | D)$-distributed, given that the proposal density q is properly adjusted and thinning of the immediate output sequence has been performed.

Note that the posterior density is required only in step 2 where we calculate the acceptance probability r for two given parameter values γ_{t-1} and γ^*. Since the two corresponding density values are divided by each other, the normalizing constant of the posterior density gets canceled out, as it depends only on the data D. Therefore, we can perform the Metropolis algorithm without even considering the normalizing constant, as long as the kernel of the posterior density can be determined. This is one reason why this algorithm has become so popular. Another reason is that due to its structural simplicity, it can be used in a vast range of situations.

3.5   Numerical Suggestions

In principle, we can directly use the Metropolis algorithm to simulate values from the joint posterior distribution of $(\lambda_1, \ldots, \lambda_m, \theta)$. In order to do so, we need to determine the proposal density q, which we can choose as a normal distribution, and derive a numerical approximation of the selection probability. The problem that we would encounter doing so is mainly that due to the possibly large number of parameters ($>m$), it might take a considerable amount of time until the Markov chain displays sufficient mixing behaviour. In addition, the acceptance rate (defined as the rate of actual parameter changes in step 3 in relation to M) would generally be dissatisfyingly low and also lead to high autocorrelation in the output sequence. Of course, one could adjust thinning of the Markov chain to overcome this problem, while further increasing the running time of the algorithm.

Instead it is preferable to change the simulation scheme using again the distinction of lifetime and birth process parameters. The proposition below shows how the posterior density can be decomposed in an important special case. Simulating according to this decomposition reduces the complexity of the posterior density, while simultaneously decreasing running time and increasing the quality of the resulting markov chain.

Proposition 3.2 *Let* $\lambda_1, \ldots, \lambda_m, \theta$ *be a priori independent and uniformly distributed on their respective parameter spaces. Then*

(1)   The marginal posterior density of θ *is given as*

$$\pi(\theta|D) \propto \prod_{i=1}^{n} f(y_i|\theta) \prod_{k=1}^{m} p_k(\theta)^{-(n_k+1)}$$

   and

(2) λ_k is conditionally Gamma distributed given θ a posteriori:

$$\lambda_k|\theta, D \sim \text{Ga}(n_k + 1, (t_k - s_k)p_k(\theta)), \quad k = 1, \ldots, m.$$

Figure 3.3 illustrates the simulation scheme according to Proposition 3.2. Specifically, we first exclusively consider the marginal posterior distribution of θ given the data D and draw from it using the Metropolis algorithm. Once the (thinned) sequence $\theta^1, \ldots, \theta^M$ is drawn, we use the conditional posterior distribution of λ_k for

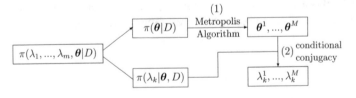

Fig. 3.3   Simulation scheme for drawing from the posterior distribution

each $k = 1, \ldots, m$, and draw from it random realizations λ_k^j for given θ^j using the conditional conjugacy. This way we obtain a sequence $(\lambda_1^j, \ldots, \lambda_m^j, \theta^j)$, of which every element has approximately joint distribution $\pi(\lambda_1, \ldots, \lambda_m, \theta | D)$.

In Appendix D, we provide an implementation of this numerical procedure in R for a simulated dataset.

3.5.1 Numerical Determination of the Selection Probability

When implementing the likelihood function, the selection probability is required. There are only some special cases for which the selection probability can be expressed in closed-form. As a general alternative, they can be numerically approximated. Having a sufficiently fast approximation is important, since when performing an MCMC algorithm, it needs to be calculated a considerable number of times.

Consider a birth period (s, t) with constant birth intensity λ. The individual selection probability for a unit from this period is given as

$$
\begin{aligned}
p(\theta) &= P(t^L \leq b^* + y^* \leq t^R | \theta, b \in (s, t)) \\[4pt]
&= \int_s^t (F(t^R - b | \theta) - F(t^L - b | \theta)) \cdot g(b | \lambda) db \\[4pt]
&= \frac{1}{t - s} \int_s^t F(t^R - b | \theta) - F(t^L - b | \theta) db \\[4pt]
&= \frac{1}{t - s} \left(\int_s^t F(t^R - b | \theta) db - \int_s^t F(t^L - b | \theta) db \right) \\[4pt]
&\overset{(1)}{=} \frac{1}{t - s} \left(\int_{s+(t^R - t^L)}^{t+(t^R - t^L)} F(t^L - b | \theta) db - \int_s^t F(t^L - b | \theta) db \right) \\[4pt]
&\overset{(2)}{=} \frac{1}{t - s} \left(\int_t^{t+(t^R - t^L)} F(t^L - b | \theta) db - \int_s^{s+(t^R - t^L)} F(t^L - b | \theta) db \right)
\end{aligned}
$$

In this derivation, step (1) uses the substitution $b \to b + (t^R - t^L)$ by which the same integrands result. Step (2) uses the fact that the intervals of the integrals in the step above overlap and thus the respective subintegrals get canceled out.

By this calculation, we have simplified the integral on (s, t) to two integrals over subintervals of length $t^R - t^L$ which may be considerably smaller. Therefore, conventional approximation of these two integrals can yield a fast approximation of $p(\theta)$. In the considered model with piecewise constant birth intensity, this approximation is carried out for each birth period $k = 1, \ldots, m$.

3.5.2 Tuning the Metropolis Algorithm

When using an MCMC algorithm, the general quality of the resulting sequence is judged on the basis of a few essential criteria, which can be checked with marginal trace and autocorrelation plots (see Robert and Casella (2004)). First of all, the transitioning behaviour through the parameter space for each component is supposed to display no ostensible systematics and to roughly cover the whole parameter range with substantial posterior probability mass. This includes that the sequence does not display periodic movements, i.e. it does not remain for a number of steps within certain parameter ranges between which it alternates. Second, the sequence should ideally depict stationary behaviour, because the approximation is valid only if the Markov chain has attained its limiting distribution. Third, the component-wise autocorrelation of the sequence is supposed to be insignificant. This property is important in order to enable valid standard error estimation. These qualitative properties can be achieved by a number of essential features.

As the marginal distribution of the chain elements converges to the target distribution, the most obvious choice is to increase the sequence length M. If the posterior distribution is well-defined and the algorithm correctly implemented, this will eventually ensure that after sufficiently many steps the chain elements are marginally distributed as desired. Similarly, excluding a number of early simulated values, i.e. by setting a burn-in size of simulated values that are discarded later, avoids considering non-convergent elements. Finally, it is important to address the autocorrelation between chain elements, which is a natural consequence of the algorithm. In general, one can choose a thinning rate $\tau \geq 1$ by which every τ-th element of the simulated chain is retained, while all other values are discarded.

3.6 Application

In the German company dataset, which is introduced in Chapter 1, companies are sampled if and only if they become insolvent during the time span of data collection, which was from September 2013 to March 2014. We restrict our attention to all companies formed after 2000, which yields $n = 4139$ observations. Double-truncation occurs naturally in this sampling scheme, since the public announcements of company insolvencies are available for the limited time span of roughly two weeks. It can be seen from the histogram of observed births (see Fig. 3.4) that truncation causes a severe distortion of the birth distribution because it is known that there is not such a substantial change in the birth intensity in the population as the histogram depicts.

We first consider the birth interval [2000, 2013.67], which we partition into the birth periods [2000, 2008) and [2008, 2013.67]. For the latent lifetimes, we assume an exponential distribution with parameter θ. The birth periods are equipped with two constant birth intensities λ_1 and λ_2, so that we altogether have $m + 1 = 3$ parameters in this model.

Fig. 3.4 Histogram of the observed births in the insolvency dataset

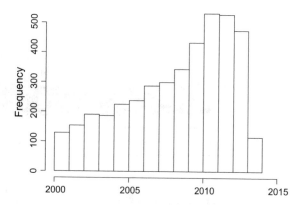

Using the described simulation scheme, we estimate the parameters of the latent lifetime distribution and the birth process (see Fig. 3.5). Despite the noticeable skew in the marginal trace plots for λ_1 and λ_2, the result does not indicate essential flaws. Here and in the analyses below, we have used $M = 5000$, burn-in size 200 and thinning rate $\tau = 20$ in the final simulation which is run after pre-adjustment of the proposal variance via preliminary shorter simulation runs (see Roberts and Rosenthal (2001) and Haario et al. (2001)).

We obtain $\widehat{\lambda}_1 = 11,399$ and $\widehat{\lambda}_2 = 15,597$, meaning that between years 2000 and 2008 roughly 11,400 companies have been founded in Germany per year, increasing to about 15,600 per year afterwards. The estimated lifetime parameter $\widehat{\theta} = 0.057$ implies that the estimated mean lifetime of a single company until insolvency is about $1/0.057 \approx 17.5$ years.

For checking the validity of the used model, we perform a number of posterior predictive checks, by which the observed characteristics of the data are compared to those implied by the fitted model (see Gelman et al. (1996)). Specifically, we use the posterior distribution to simulate pseudo-datasets subject to the double-truncation. Generating these datasets includes drawing random population sizes N_k, random births b_i^* and lifetimes y_i^* and subjecting these to the selection mechanism $t^L \leq b_i^* + y_i^* \leq t^R$, which results in random replicated datasets D_j^{rep} for each $j \in \{1, ..., M\}$.

For each of these simulated datasets, we can determine basic characteristics such as the mean and variance of the lifetimes. Combining each of these values, we implicitly estimate a probabilty distribution and confidence interval of the respective test quantity T, which in turn indicates whether the observed value $T(D)$ is plausible under the fitted model. We consider the fitted model plausible (with respect to T), if the observed value $T(D)$ lies within the confidence interval. Equivalently, the corresponding p-values should not be below $\alpha_C/2$ or above $1 - \alpha_C/2$, where α_C denotes the desired significance level. Vice versa, if an observed value $T(D)$ is not located in the confidence interval, this indicates that the model is not suitable for inference concerning the test quantity T. In this manner, we can use any test quantity T that we find important for inferential purposes.

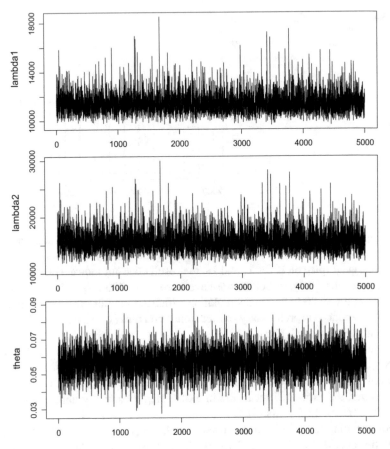

Fig. 3.5 MCMC output for the model with $y^* \sim \text{Exp}(\theta)$ and birth periods $[2000, 2008)$ and $[2008, 2013.67]$

Table 3.1 Posterior predictive check for the model with $y^* \sim \text{Exp}(\theta)$ and birth periods $[2000, 2008)$ and $[2008, 2013.67]$

Test quantity	Observed value	Confidence interval (95%)	p-value
Mean of y	5.73	(5.57, 5.90)	0.47
Median of y	4.94	(4.79, 5.22)	0.29
Variance of y	12.52	(14.09, 15.12)	0.00
Interquartile range of y	5.51	(5.96, 6.47)	0.00

From Table 3.1, we can see that the observed variance and interquartile range of y are not plausible under the fitted model, while the mean and median are. As a consequence, the model assumptions are not optimal and we may seek for model improvements.

It is possible that assuming exponentially distributed lifetimes is too strict. Instead we consider the Gamma distribution with density function

Table 3.2 Estimation results for the model with $y^* \sim Ga(\alpha, \beta)$ and birth periods [2000, 2004), [2004, 2008), [2008, 2012) and [2012, 2013.67]

		Parameter	Estimate	SE
Birth intensities	2000–2004	λ_1	10,180	926.600
	2004–2008	λ_2	7048	282.345
	2008–2012	λ_3	7403	377.467
	2012–2013.67	λ_4	8133	738.161
Lifetime distribution		α	1.96	0.095
		β	0.31	0.025

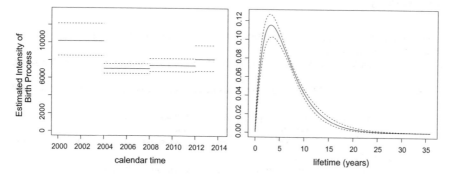

Fig. 3.6 Estimated birth intensities and lifetime density function

$$f(y|\alpha, \beta) = \frac{\beta^\alpha}{\Gamma(\alpha)} y^{\alpha-1} e^{-\beta y},$$

where $\alpha > 0$ and $\beta > 0$. The same birth period setting is used as before and the prior distribution is again assumed to be uniform. This model results in $(\widehat{\alpha}, \widehat{\beta}) = (1.71, 0.22)$ and $(\widehat{\lambda}_1, \widehat{\lambda}_2) = (7590, 8956)$. Based on this point estimate, approximately 7590 companies were founded per year between 2000 and 2008, and 8956 per year between 2008 and September 2013. The mean lifetime of these companies is estimated to be $1.71/0.22 \approx 7.72$ years.

A posterior predictive check in the same manner as for the previous model (omitted here) indicates that the fitted model seems questionable, as the observed median lifetime and the interquartile range are not within 95% intervals. Therefore, we make one final adjustment to the model and change the birth period setting by further partitioning the birth interval into 4 periods (see Table 3.2).

The trace plots of the simulated Markov chain have been checked for convergence and stationarity. The results (see Table 3.2 and Fig. 3.6) indicate that there has been a significant change in the birth process throughout the years 2000–2014. The estimated mean lifetime in the latent population is about 6.3 years with a standard deviation of about 4.5 years. Judging from the posterior predictive checks that have been carried out (see Table 3.3) this model seems plausible for the considered dataset.

Table 3.3 Posterior predictive check for the model with $y^* \sim Ga(\alpha, \beta)$ and birth periods [2000, 2004), [2004, 2008), [2008, 2012) and [2012, 2013.67]

Test quantity	Observed value	Confidence interval (95%)	p-value
Mean of y	5.73	(5.58, 5.88)	0.49
Median of y	4.94	(4.89, 5.28)	0.07
Variance of y	12.52	(11.50, 12.65)	0.93
Interquartile range of y	5.51	(5.03, 5.55)	0.95

References

Bayarri MJ, DeGroot MH (1987) Bayesian analysis of selection models. J R Stat Soc Ser D (The Statistician) 36:137–146

Efron B, Petrosian V (1999) Nonparametric methods for doubly truncated data. J Am Stat Assoc 94(447):824–834

Emura T, Konno Y (2012) Multivariate normal distribution approaches for dependently truncated data. Stat Pap 53:133–149

Emura T, Hu Y-H, Konno Y (2017) Asymptotic inference for maximum likelihood estimators under the special exponential family with double-truncation. Stat Pap 58(3):877–909

Gelman A, Meng X-L, Stern HS (1996) Posterior predictive assessment of model fitness via realized discrepancies. Stat Sinica 6:733–807

Haario H, Saksman E, Tamminen J (2001) An Adaptive metropolis algorithm. Bernoulli 7(2):223–242

Hu Y-H, Emura T (2015) Maximum likelihood estimation for a special exponential family under random double-truncation. Comput Stat 30:1199–1229. https://doi.org/10.1007/s00180-015-0564-z

Kalbfleisch JD, Lawless JF (1989) Inference based on retrospective ascertainment: an analysis of the data on transfusion-related aids. J Am Stat Assoc 84:360–372

Lawless J, Kalbfleisch JD (1992) Some issues in the collection and analysis of field reliability data, pp 141–152. Kluwer Academic Publishers, Dordrecht/Boston/London

Lee J, Berger JO (2001) Semiparametric bayesian analysis of selection models. J Am Stat Assoc 96:1397–1409

Robert CP, Casella G (2004) Monte Carlo statistical methods, Springer

Roberts GO, Rosenthal JS (2001) Optimal scaling for various metropolis-hastings algorithms. Stat Sci 16(4):351–367

Sanathanan L (1972) Estimating the size of a multinomial population. Ann Math Stat 43:142–152

Sanathanan L (1977) Estimating the size of a truncated sample. J Am Stat Assoc 72:669–672

Scheike TH, Keiding N (2006) Design and analysis of time-to-pregnancy. Stat Methods Med Res 15:127–140

Shen P-S (2017) Pseudo maximum likelihood estimation for the Cox model with doubly truncated data. Stat Pap. https://doi.org/10.1007/s00362-016-0870-8

Tierney L (1994) Markov chains for exploring posterior distributions. Ann Stat 22:1701–1728

Wang M-C (1989) A semiparametric model for randomly truncated data. J Am Stat Assoc 84:742–748

West M (1994) Discovery sampling and selection models. In: Gupta SS, Berger JO (eds) Statistical decision theory and related topics V, pp 221–235

West M (1996) Inference in successive sampling discovery models. J Econometr 75:217–238

Chapter 4
Nonparametric Inference for Double-Truncation

Abstract In this chapter, the nonparametric maximum likelihood estimate (NPMLE) for random variables under double-truncation is presented. In contrast to parametric approaches, no specific distributional assumptions are made, and it is described how the estimator originally derived in Efron and Petrosian (J Am Stat Assoc 94(447):824–834, 1999) is defined and motivated. It turns out that the solution to the estimation problem can be regarded as a fixed-point. We reproduce key ideas from Shen (Ann Inst Stat Math 62:835–853, 2010) who offered more extensive explanations and important insights on the likelihood alternatives. In addition, theoretical properties of the procedure including consistency are stated. The method is applied to the Equipment-S dataset.

Keywords Nonparametric inference · Double-truncation ·
Likelihood construction · Conditional likelihood · Observational data · Bootstrap

4.1 Introduction

For the nonparametric approach, the general intent is to impose as few assumptions on the involved distributions as possible. In particular, no parametric distribution families are taken as a modelling basis. For doubly truncated observations, we essentially deal with three random variables: two random truncation variables U^* and V^*, and one variable of interest Y^* which is observed if and only if $U^* \leq Y^* \leq V^*$. We derive estimators of the corresponding distribution functions F of Y^* and K of (U^*, V^*), where estimating F is of primary interest. Note that we explicitly consider the *joint* distribution of U^* and V^* in order to allow them to be dependent. In addition, it is generally assumed that Y^* is independent of the truncation variables. If this were not fulfilled, consistent estimation of F would be difficult in general (see Tsai 1990). Efron and Petrosian (1999), Martin and Betensky (2005) and Shen (2010) discussed the importance of the independence assumption in nonparametric inference, and developed nonparametric tests to verify the assumption.

   In contrast to parametric approaches, identifiability is a more delicate issue in the nonparametric framework. If, for instance, only some subset of the support of Y^* were

© The Author(s), under exclusive license to Springer Nature Singapore Pte Ltd. 2019
A. Dörre and T. Emura, *Analysis of Doubly Truncated Data*, JSS Research
Series in Statistics, https://doi.org/10.1007/978-981-13-6241-5_4

63

covered by the range of (U^*, V^*), one would be unable to collect any information on the remaining support of Y^*. Identifiability of Y^* is thus generally limited to the observed support of Y^* for technical reasons.

Even though the distributions are usually modelled as continuous, their estimators are chosen as discrete distributions whose support is given by the observed data points. Note that by this choice the estimation problem is actually transformed into a parametric (multinomial) one where each observed data point is assigned to a density parameter. In this sense, the model is parametric, but with indefinite dimension depending on the sample size.

The basis of the presented methods can be traced back to Turnbull (1976), after which Efron and Petrosian (1999) specifically derived the nonparametric maximum likelihood estimator (NPMLE) for doubly truncated data. Shen (2010) investigated further fundamental properties of the NPMLE, which is the main reference for this chapter. An explicit formula for the standard error of the estimated distribution function was developed in Emura et al. (2015). Resampling-based methods for determining standard errors and confidence intervals for the estimated distribution function were also considered in Moreira and Uña-Álvarez (2010), where a simple bootstrap method is suggested, and in Emura et al. (2015) who employed a jackknife method.

In this chapter, first the rationale of a nonparametric estimator is illustrated in Sect. 4.2, after which in Sect. 4.3 a more formal perspective is taken along with a practical algorithm. Section 4.4 contains the fundamental asymptotic properties and describes how standard errors can be approximated. Finally, in Sect. 4.5, we demonstrate the method on the Equipment-S dataset.

4.2 Heuristic Derivation of the NPMLE of f

In this section, we provide a heuristic deviation of the NPMLE based on a conditional likelihood function. We also provide an illustrative example to compute the NPMLE.

The selection criterion underlying doubly truncated data is that a unit is observed if and only if $U^* \leq Y^* \leq V^*$, which is clearly fulfilled for all observed data points (u_i, v_i, y_i), $i = 1, \ldots, n$. We define the corresponding observed region $R_i := [u_i, v_i]$ for each unit $i = 1, \ldots, n$, which is the range in which any $y \in R_i$ would have been observed. Suppose that $F(y) := \mathrm{P}(Y^* \leq y)$ is the true distribution function of Y^* (before truncation) and $f(y) := dF(y)/dy$ the corresponding true density function on the lifetime support $\mathcal{Y}$. The conditional density of Y^* given $Y^* \in R_i$ is

$$f(y|R_i) = \begin{cases} f(y)/F_i & y \in R_i \\ 0 & \text{else} \end{cases} \tag{4.1}$$

Table 4.1 Illustrative doubly truncated data example from Efron and Petrosian (1999)

y_i	$R_i = [u_i, v_i]$
0.75	[0.4, 2.0]
1.25	[0.8, 1.8]
1.50	[0.0, 2.3]
1.05	[0.3, 1.4]
2.40	[1.1, 3.0]
2.50	[2.3, 3.4]
2.25	[1.3, 2.6]

where

$$F_i := \int_{R_i} f(y)dy$$

is the probability mass corresponding to the region R_i for given f. We can use this conditional density function for estimating f. Pursuing the nonparametric paradigm, we restrict our attention to all discrete distributions having probability mass on the observed set of values $(y_1, \ldots, y_n)$. Thus we represent the distribution of Y^* by a vector $f = (f_1, \ldots, f_n)$ with $\sum f_i = 1$. The probability masses F_i are correspondingly defined as subsums of f in this framework. For the derivation, we follow the illustrative example provided in Efron and Petrosian (1999) that consists of $n = 7$ observations (see Table 4.1).

Conditional on R_i, the probability of observing unit i can be determined as

$$F_i = P(i \text{ is observed} | R_i) = \sum_{j=1}^{n} I(u_i \leq y_j \leq v_i) \cdot f_j$$

for given f. We define the $n \times n$ indicator matrix J as $J_{ij} := I(u_i \leq y_j \leq v_i)$. Based on J, all conditional selection probabilities given the respective observed regions R_i can be written as

$$F = Jf. \tag{4.2}$$

In the illustrative example, we obtain

$$J = \begin{pmatrix} 1 & 1 & 1 & 1 & 0 & 0 & 0 \\ 0 & 1 & 1 & 1 & 0 & 0 & 0 \\ 1 & 1 & 1 & 1 & 0 & 0 & 1 \\ 1 & 1 & 0 & 1 & 0 & 0 & 0 \\ 0 & 1 & 1 & 0 & 1 & 1 & 1 \\ 0 & 0 & 0 & 0 & 1 & 1 & 0 \\ 0 & 0 & 1 & 0 & 1 & 1 & 1 \end{pmatrix}$$

The first row $(1, 1, 1, 1, 0, 0, 0)$ of J, for instance, represents the fact that precisely the units 1, 2, 3 and 4 would have been observed in the first region R_1. If $f = (1/n, \ldots, 1/n)$, the conditional probability of observing unit 1 is thus $4/7 \approx 0.57$.

Combining the conditional probabilities according to Eq. (4.1), we obtain the likelihood function

$$L(f|J) = \prod_{i=1}^{n} \frac{f_i}{F_i} = \prod_{i=1}^{n} \frac{f_i}{\sum_{m=1}^{n} J_{im} f_m},$$

defined for vectors $f \in [0, 1]^n$ with $\sum f_i = 1$ conditional on the indicator matrix J. The log-likelihood function can thus be determined as

$$\ln L(f|J) = \sum_{i=1}^{n} \ln f_i - \sum_{i=1}^{n} \ln F_i = \sum_{i=1}^{n} \ln f_i - \sum_{i=1}^{n} \ln \left(\sum_{m=1}^{n} J_{im} f_m \right).$$

For obtaining the maximum likelihood solution, we calculate the first derivative with respect to f_i,

$$\frac{\partial \ln L}{\partial f_i} = \frac{1}{f_i} - \sum_{j=1}^{n} \frac{J_{ji}}{\sum_{m=1}^{n} J_{jm} f_m} = \frac{1}{f_i} - \sum_{j=1}^{n} \frac{J_{ji}}{F_j},$$

by which we obtain the first-order conditions

$$\frac{1}{f_i} = \sum_{j=1}^{n} \frac{J_{ji}}{F_j} \quad \forall i = 1, \ldots, n.$$

As both sides of the equation depend on f, it constitutes a fixed-point equation (see Burden and Faires 2011) which is compactly expressed as

$$\frac{1}{f} = J^{\mathsf{T}} \frac{1}{F}. \tag{4.3}$$

This system of equations can be used to construct an iterative algorithm for determining the solution. Specifically, starting from an initial value for f, we can repeatedly use Eq. (4.2) to determine F from f, and Eq. (4.3) to determine f based on F. Once this procedure has converged to a stable point f, we have found the maximum likelihood estimate.

1. Set $f^{(0)} = (1/n, \ldots, 1/n)$ and $t := 0$.
2. Calculate $F^{(t)} = J f^{(t)}$.
3. Increase t by 1, and calculate

$$f_i^{(t)} = \left(\sum_{j=1}^n \frac{J_{ji}}{F_j^{(t-1)}} \right)^{-1} \quad \forall i = 1, \dots, n,$$

and normalize $\boldsymbol{f}^{(t)}$ so that $\sum_{i=1}^n f_i^{(t)} = 1$.

4. Repeat steps 2 and 3 until $\boldsymbol{f}^{(t)}$ is stable, i.e. stop the algorithm when $\| \boldsymbol{f}^{(t)} - \boldsymbol{f}^{(t-1)} \| < \varepsilon$ for some suitably chosen $\varepsilon > 0$ and some norm $\| \cdot \|$. Set $\widehat{\boldsymbol{f}} = \boldsymbol{f}^{(t)}$.

Based on $\widehat{\boldsymbol{f}}$, the cumulative distribution function is estimated as

$$\widehat{F}(y) = \sum_{y_i \leq y} \widehat{f_i}$$

for all $y \in \mathcal{Y}$. Efron and Petrosian (1999) showed that the NPMLE of F is equivalent to Lynden-Bell's (1971) estimator when there is no right-truncation ($V_i^* = \infty$). It is interesting to see that these fundamental statistical methodologies were developed in astronomical research.

Table 4.2 shows the first 5 iterations of this procedure for the illustrative example. Starting from the initial uniform estimate $f = (1/n, \dots, 1/n)$, which would be the nonparametric maximum likelihood estimate for non-truncated data, the density values substantially change in the first update. The subsequent iterations lead to smaller changes, until eventually the fixed-point $\widehat{f} \approx (0.14, 0.08, 0.09, 0.09, 0.18, 0.18, 0.23)$ is attained after about 20 iterations. As is apparent from Table 4.2, the value of the log-likelihood function may actually drop for some iterations before eventually approaching its maximum.

Each component of f represents the probability of observing the corresponding value y in the latent population, i.e. before truncation. Therefore, the resulting vector $\widehat{f} = (0.14, 0.08, 0.09, 0.09, 0.18, 0.18, 0.23)$ means that $y_1 = 0.75$ occurs with probability 0.14, $y_2 = 1.25$ with probability 0.08, and so on (see Fig. 4.1), while truncation leads to different sampling probabilities in the sample.

An R package *double.truncation* (Emura et al. 2019) can automatically compute the NPMLE including the estimators of f and F as well as the standard errors of F. The following R codes can be applied for analyzing the illustrative example:

Table 4.2 Density values for the first five iterations of the conditional NPMLE algorithm for the illustrative example

	f_1	f_2	f_3	f_4	f_5	f_6	f_7	$\ln L$
1	0.143	0.143	0.143	0.143	0.143	0.143	0.143	-8.88
2	0.173	0.103	0.110	0.121	0.143	0.143	0.208	-9.08
3	0.168	0.096	0.105	0.111	0.150	0.150	0.221	-8.74
4	0.161	0.092	0.102	0.106	0.157	0.157	0.225	-8.69
5	0.155	0.089	0.101	0.102	0.163	0.163	0.227	-8.68

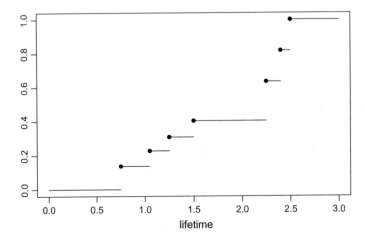

Fig. 4.1 Estimated distribution function in the illustrative example

```
library(double.truncation)
y.trunc = c(0.75, 1.25, 1.50, 1.05, 2.40, 2.50, 2.25)
u.trunc = c(0.4, 0.8, 0.0, 0.3, 1.1, 2.3, 1.3)
v.trunc = c(2.0, 1.8, 2.3, 1.4, 3.0, 3.4, 2.6)
NPMLE(u.trunc, y.trunc, v.trunc)
```

The output of the R codes show the identical results as Table 4.2.

By means of this algorithm, we obtain an estimate of the density function f without explicitly considering the distribution of either U^* or V^*, which are only indirectly considered through the indicator matrix J. Shen (2010) showed that this conditional view is sufficient for estimating f, meaning that the resulting estimator from a joint approach as outlined in Sect. 4.3 is the same as from the conditional approach above, which is true not just asymptotically, but also for finite samples (see Theorem 4.1). In the following, we reformulate the estimator from a more general perspective which also yields an estimate of the joint distribution of the truncation variables.

4.3   Joint Maximum Likelihood Estimate of f and k

In addition to f, we now consider a vector $k = (k_1, \ldots, k_n)$ containing the density values on the observed pairs (u_i, v_i), $i = 1, \ldots, n$. We maintain the definition of the indicator matrix $J_{ij} := \mathrm{I}(u_i \leq y_j \leq v_i)$ and write the joint likelihood function of the parameter vectors f and k as

$$L(f, k) = \prod_{i=1}^{n} \frac{f_i k_i}{\sum_{j=1}^{n} F_j k_j} \tag{4.4}$$

where $F_i = \sum_{j=1}^{n} J_{ij} f_j$, as before. Note that the term $\sum_{j=1}^{n} F_j k_j = \sum_{j=1}^{n} \sum_{i=1}^{n} k_j f_i J_{ji}$ in the denominator is the unconditional selection probability of any random unit in the population based on f and k. The joint NPMLE $(\widehat{f}, \widehat{k})$ is defined as the maximizing pair of the joint likelihood function $L(f, k)$. Equivalent to Eq. (4.4), we can write

$$L(f, k) = \prod_{i=1}^{n} \frac{f_i}{F_i} \times \prod_{i=1}^{n} \frac{F_i k_i}{\sum_{j=1}^{n} F_j k_j} = L_1(f) \times L_2(f, k)$$

and in doing so partition the likelihood function into a conditional and marginal part. By just using $L_1(f)$ for estimation, we obtain the nonparametric estimator of f as motivated in Sect. 4.2. In complete analogy, we can also rearrange the terms of $L(f, k)$ such thatlikelihood function!conditional

$$L(f, k) = \prod_{i=1}^{n} \frac{k_i}{K_i} \times \prod_{i=1}^{n} \frac{K_i f_i}{\sum_{j=1}^{n} K_j f_j} = L_1(k) \times L_2(k, f),$$

where $K_i = \sum_{m=1}^{n} k_m J_{mi}$ is the probability of observing the ith unit conditional on y_i, and likewise obtain a nonparametric estimator of the density function $k : \mathcal{U} \times \mathcal{V} \to \mathbb{R}_{\geq 0}$ by maximizing $L_1(k)$. This estimator fulfils the system of equations

$$\frac{1}{k_j} = \sum_{i=1}^{n} \frac{J_{ji}}{K_i} \quad \forall j = 1, \ldots, n, \tag{4.5}$$

based on which the estimate can be constructed using an iterative algorithm in analogous fashion to Sect. 4.2 for $\widehat{f}$. Note that in this system of equations, the index pair (j, i) is used on J whereas (i, j) is used in the corresponding formulas for $\widehat{f}$.

It is an interesting question how the two estimators $\widehat{f}$ and $\widehat{k}$ obtained by respectively using $L_1(f)$ and $L_1(k)$ are related to the maximizer of the joint likelihood function L in Eq. (4.4), because we might lose information and efficiency compared to the joint MLE if these estimators differ (see Wang et al. 1986; Wang 1987). Shen (2010) shows that they are in fact identical and argued that the nonparametric estimators $\widehat{f}$ and $\widehat{k}$ immediately yield the nonparametric estimators of the distribution functions of Y^* and (U^*, V^*) as well. In particular, Shen (2010) argues that the joint MLE is obtained as the solution to the following two equations:

$$\widehat{F}(y) = \left[\sum_{i=1}^{n} \frac{1}{\widehat{K}(Y_i, \infty) - \widehat{K}(Y_i, Y_i)} \right]^{-1} \sum_{i=1}^{n} \frac{I(Y_i \leq y)}{\widehat{K}(Y_i, \infty) - \widehat{K}(Y_i, Y_i)} \tag{4.6}$$

$$\widehat{K}(u, v) = \left[\sum_{i=1}^{n} \frac{1}{\widehat{F}(V_i) - \widehat{F}(U_i-)} \right]^{-1} \sum_{i=1}^{n} \frac{I(U_i \leq u, V_i \leq v)}{\widehat{F}(V_i) - \widehat{F}(U_i-)} \tag{4.7}$$

Theorem 4.1 *Let* $\widehat{F}_{NP}(y) = \sum_{i=1}^{n} \widehat{f}_i I(Y_i \leq y)$ *and* $\widehat{K}_{NP}(u, v) = \sum_{i=1}^{n} \widehat{k}_i I(U_i \leq u, V_i \leq v)$ *be the estimated distribution functions according to the maximizers* $\widehat{f}$ *and* $\widehat{k}$ *of the conditional likelihood functions* $L_1(f)$ *and* $L_1(k)$, *respectively. Then*

(a) $\widehat{f}$ *and* $\widehat{k}$ *are the NPMLEs of the full joint likelihood function* $L(f, k)$ *and*
(b) $\widehat{F}(y) = \widehat{F}_{NP}(y)$ *and* $\widehat{K}(u, v) = \widehat{K}_{NP}(u, v)$ *are the NPMLEs of* F *and* K, *respectively.*

Proof This proof is due to Shen (2010).

As argued in Wang (1987), the estimators $\widehat{f}$ and $\widehat{k}$ need to fulfil

$$\frac{\widehat{F}_j \widehat{k}_j}{\sum_{i=1}^{n} \widehat{F}_i \widehat{k}_i} = \frac{1}{n} \quad \text{and} \quad \frac{\widehat{K}_j \widehat{f}_j}{\sum_{i=1}^{n} \widehat{K}_i \widehat{f}_i} = \frac{1}{n} \quad \forall j = 1, \ldots, n \tag{4.8}$$

in order to be the maximizing pair of the full joint likelihood L. Now for any $j = 1, \ldots, n$, let $\widehat{f}_{wj} = [\sum_{i=1}^{n} \frac{1}{\widehat{K}_i}]^{-1} \frac{1}{\widehat{K}_j}$ and $\widehat{k}_{wj} = [\sum_{i=1}^{n} \frac{1}{\widehat{F}_i}]^{-1} \frac{1}{\widehat{F}_j}$. It can be directly shown that $\widehat{f}_{wj}$ and $\widehat{k}_{wj}$ fulfil Eq. (4.8) and thus are the maximizers of the joint likelihood function. Note that by definition of $\widehat{f}_{wj}$ and due to Eq. (4.5), it also holds that

$$\left[\sum_{i=1}^{n} J_{ij} \frac{1}{\sum_{m=1}^{n} \widehat{f}_{wm} J_{im}} \right]^{-1} = \left[\sum_{i=1}^{n} J_{ij} \frac{1}{\sum_{m=1}^{n} (\sum_{i=1}^{n} \frac{1}{\widehat{K}_i})^{-1} \frac{1}{\widehat{K}_m} \cdot J_{im}} \right]^{-1}$$

$$= \left(\sum_{i=1}^{n} \frac{1}{\widehat{K}_i} \right)^{-1} \left[\sum_{i=1}^{n} J_{ij} \frac{1}{\sum_{m=1}^{n} \frac{1}{\widehat{K}_m} J_{im}} \right]^{-1}$$

$$= \left(\sum_{i=1}^{n} \frac{1}{\widehat{K}_i} \right)^{-1} \left[\sum_{i=1}^{n} J_{ij} \widehat{k}_i \right]$$

$$= \left(\sum_{i=1}^{n} \frac{1}{\widehat{K}_i} \right)^{-1} \frac{1}{\widehat{K}_j}$$

$$= \widehat{f}_{wj}.$$

It can be similarly proven that $\widehat{k}_{wj} = [\sum_{i=1}^{n} J_{ji} \frac{1}{\sum_{m=1}^{n} \widehat{k}_{wm} J_{mi}}]^{-1}$. In other words, the maximizers of $L(f, k)$ also fulfil the characterization of the conditional estimators. Since the components of $\widehat{f}$ and $\widehat{k}$ add up to 1, it follows that $\widehat{f}_j = \widehat{f}_{wj}$ and $\widehat{k}_j = \widehat{k}_{wj}$ for every $j = 1, \ldots, n$. Therefore, assertion (a) is proven. It is also implied that

$$\widehat{f}_j = \left[\sum_{i=1}^{n} \frac{1}{\widehat{K}_i}\right]^{-1} \frac{1}{\widehat{K}_j} \tag{4.9}$$

$$\widehat{k}_j = \left[\sum_{i=1}^{n} \frac{1}{\widehat{F}_i}\right]^{-1} \frac{1}{\widehat{F}_j} \tag{4.10}$$

for all $j = 1, \ldots, n$.

For (b), note that $\widehat{K}(Y_i, \infty) - \widehat{K}(Y_i, Y_i)$ is equal to the marginal probability of observing Y_i for given estimate $\widehat{K}$. Likewise, $\widehat{F}(V_i) - \widehat{F}(U_i-)$ is the marginal probability of observing (U_i, V_i) for given $\widehat{F}$. Thus we have $\widehat{K}_i = \widehat{K}(Y_i, \infty) - \widehat{K}(Y_i, Y_i)$ and $\widehat{F}_i = \widehat{F}(V_i) - \widehat{F}(U_i-)$.

Plugging this into Eqs. (4.6) and (4.7) shows that Eqs. (4.9) and (4.10) are fulfilled and therefore (b) is true. □

This proof also shows that the NPMLE can be obtained using Eqs. (4.9) and (4.10) as in the following iterative algorithm:

1. Set $f^{(0)} = (1/n, \ldots, 1/n)$ and $t := 0$.
2. Calculate $F^{(t)} = J f^{(t)}$ and determine

$$k_j^{(t+1)} = \left[\sum_{i=1}^{n} \frac{1}{F_i^{(t)}}\right]^{-1} \frac{1}{F_j^{(t)}}, \quad j = 1, \ldots, n$$

3. Calculate $K^{(t+1)} = J^{\mathsf{T}} k^{(t+1)}$ and determine

$$f_j^{(t+1)} = \left[\sum_{i=1}^{n} \frac{1}{K_i^{(t+1)}}\right]^{-1} \frac{1}{K_j^{(t+1)}}, \quad j = 1, \ldots, n$$

   and increase t by 1.
4. Repeat steps 2 and 3 until f and k are stable.

Note that by steps 2 and 3 in the algorithm, we implicitly consider a function $(f^{(t)}, k^{(t)}) \mapsto (f^{(t+1)}, k^{(t+1)})$. Convergence of the algorithm is equivalent to $(f^{(t+1)}, k^{(t+1)}) = (f^{(t)}, k^{(t)})$ because updating f and k has to be invariant when f and k are stable. We can thus consider the estimator as a solution to this fixed-point problem (see Burden and Faires 2011), if it exists.

4.4 Asymptotic Properties and Bootstrap Approximation

For any given random variable X, define $a_X := \inf\{x | F^X(x) > 0\}$ and $b_X := \inf\{x | F^X(x) = 1\}$, so that the support of X is (a_X, b_X). We impose the following assumption:

(A) It holds that $a_{U^*} \leq a_{Y^*} \leq a_{V^*}$ and $b_{U^*} \leq b_{Y^*} \leq b_{V^*}$.

Assumption (A) means that the support of Y^* has to be completely observable under the distribution of (U^*, V^*) and vice versa. When this is true, both distribution functions F and K are identifiable with respect to the truncated sample (see Woodroofe 1985). Under two additional regularity conditions (see Shen 2010 for details), the following result shows that F is also consistently estimated.

Theorem 4.2 *Let a_F, $\tau \in [0, \infty)$ be such that $F(v) - F(u-) > \delta > 0$ for $[u, v] \subseteq [a_F, \tau]$. Moreover, assume that (a) $\int_{a_F}^{\tau} F(dx)/[K(x, \infty) - K(x, x)] < \infty$ and (b) $[K(dx, \infty) - K(dx, dx)]/F(dx)$ is uniformly bounded on $[a_F, \tau]$. Then the NPMLE $\widehat{F}$ is uniformly consistent on $[a_F, \tau]$.*

Proof For the proof, see Shen (2010). □

Shen (2010) also proves that $\sqrt{n}(\widehat{F}(t) - F(t))$ is asymptotically normal in an interval $[a_F, \tau]$, given certain regularity conditions which are usually fulfilled. Motivated by these results, we approximate confidence intervals using a bootstrap approximation as suggested in Moreira and Uña-Álvarez (2010). In particular, we draw B random subsamples $(U_i^{(b)}, V_i^{(b)}, Y_i^{(b)})$, $i = 1, \ldots, n$, $b = 1, \ldots, B$, each having size n from the data and calculate the NPMLEs. This yields a sequence of nonparametric estimates, which represent an empirical approximation of the true sampling distribution of the NPMLE $\widehat{F}$ when B is sufficiently large. Consequently, quantiles can directly be determined and used as pointwise confidence intervals. Specifically, we suggest using a predetermined grid of the observed range of Y^* and to calculate $\widehat{F}^{(b)}(y) = \sum_{i=1}^{n} \widehat{f}_i^{(b)} I(Y_i^{(b)} \leq y)$ for each bootstrap sample.

There are different options to compute the variance estimator of the NPMLE and the pointwise confidence interval of F beyond the simple bootstrap. Emura et al. (2015) suggested the asymptotic variance formula and the jackknife method. According to the simulation studies of Emura et al. (2015), the jackknife has the smallest bias. In terms of mean squared error of variance estimation, the bootstrap is the best for small samples, while the asymptotic variance method tends to be the best for large samples. However, the numerical performance of these three methods are comparable since they estimate the same quantities.

4.5 Application

We apply the NPMLE on the Equipment-S dataset from Ye and Tang (2015) (see Chap. 1). For an R implementation of this application, see Appendix E. After eliminating all units with installation date after the year 1996, $n = 161$ observations out of 174 remain. The units installed after the year 1996 correspond to the smallest values of U^* and are excluded since they seem to considerably distort the estimation of the distribution of the truncation variables. If more observations were available for dates after 1996, this step would be unnecessary.

Applying the algorithm from Sect. 4.3 yields the estimates $\widehat{f}$ and $\widehat{k}$ from which we deduce the distribution of the lifetimes (see Fig. 4.2) as well as the median lifetime of 20.4 years for individual units, respectively. Note that lifetimes larger than 35 can not be recorded by definition of the observation window. We thus effectively estimate the conditional distribution function $F(y)/F(35)$ and can make no conclusions on the survival behaviour for $y > 35$.

Furthermore, one may be interested in the distribution of the installation dates of the units. This can be immediately achieved because the individual installation dates are given by $s_i = 1996 - u_i, i = 1, \ldots, n$, and thus the distribution of s_i is the same

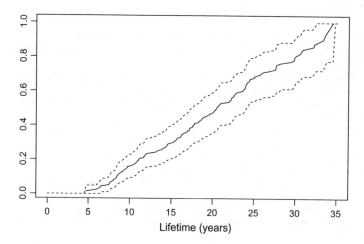

Fig. 4.2 Estimated cumulative distribution function of the units' lifetimes including 90% bootstrap pointwise confidence bounds

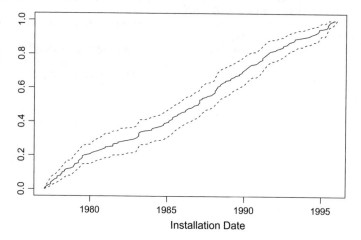

Fig. 4.3 Estimated cumulative distribution function of the units' installation dates including 90% bootstrap pointwise confidence bounds

as for u_i after appropriate mapping. Since for this dataset $V^* - U^* \equiv const = 16$, the estimated density value at any s_i is $\widehat{k}_i$. Consequently, we estimate the distribution of the installation dates (see Fig. 4.3).

It can be seen that both the lifetime and installation date distribution are roughly linear. This means that units are installed with a relatively constant rate during the years. Similarly, the units fail at some random lifetime between 5 and 35 years, with no decided tendency towards smaller or larger lifetimes.

References

Burden RL, Faires JD (2011) Numerical analysis, 9th edn. Cengage Learning

Efron B, Petrosian V (1999) Nonparametric methods for doubly truncated data. J Am Stat Assoc 94(447):824–834

Emura T, Konno Y, Michimae H (2015) Statistical inference based on the nonparametric maximum likelihood estimator under double-truncation. Lifetime Data Anal 21:397–418

Emura T, Hu YH, Huang CY (2019) double.truncation: analysis of doubly-truncated data, R package version 1.4. CRAN

Lynden-Bell D (1971) A method of allowing for known observational selection in small samples applied to 3CR quasars. Mon Not R Astron Soc 155:95–118

Martin EC, Betensky RA (2005) Testing quasi-independence of failure and truncation times via conditional Kendall's tau. J Am Stat Assoc 100:484–492

Moreira C, Uña-Álvarez J (2010) Bootstrapping the NPMLE for doubly truncated data. J Nonparametr Stat 22:567–583

Shen P-S (2010) Nonparametric analysis of doubly truncated data. Ann Inst Stat Math 62:835–853

Tsai W-Y (1990) Testing the assumption of independence of truncation time and failure time. Biometrika 77(1):169–177

Turnbull BW (1976) The empirical distribution function with arbitrarily grouped, censored and truncated data. J R Stat Soc Ser B Methodol 38(3):290–295

Wang M-C, Jewell NP, Tsai W-Y (1986) Asymptotic properties of the product limit estimate under random truncation. Ann Stat 14(4):1597–1605

Wang M-C (1987) Product limit estimates: a generalized maximum likelihood study. Commun Stat Theory Methods 16(11):3117–3132

Woodroofe M (1985) Estimating a distribution function with truncated data. Ann Stat 13(1):163–177

Ye Z-S, Tang L-C (2015) Augmenting the unreturned for field data with information on returned failures only. Technometrics. https://doi.org/10.1080/00401706.2015.1093033

Chapter 5
Linear Regression Under Random Double-Truncation

Abstract We investigate the well-known linear regression model under double-truncation, i.e. the response variable is subjected to random double-truncation. It is argued that the conventional OLS estimator is not valid when truncation is present. Instead, a fundamental property of the regression equation is used to construct a non-parametric plug-in-type estimator. The method is based on the NPMLE which is treated in Chap. 4 (see also Efron and Petrosian in J Am Stat Assoc 94(447):824–834, 1999; Shen in Ann Inst Stat Math 62:835–853, 2010). It is described how the estimator and related aspects can be estimated and how standard errors can be approximated via a bootstrap procedure. Asymptotic properties including consistency and asymptotic normality are stated. The method is finally applied to a dataset of German insolvent companies which was introduced in Chap. 1.

Keywords Non-parametric inference · Double-truncation · Linear regression · Observational data · Bootstrap

5.1 Introduction

In many practical situations where truncation occurs, covariates are measured along the response variable and one wishes to assess their respective impact. In this chapter, we investigate the linear regression model, for which the response variable is subjected to random double-truncation. For this, we employ the non-parametric maximum likelihood estimator (NPMLE) explained in Chap. 4 (Shen 2010; Efron and Petrosian 1999; Emura et al. 2015) in order to derive estimators of the regression coefficients. Note that we specifically consider truncation of the response variable, i.e. truncation potentially occurs once the value of the response variable is realized. The linear regression model under left-truncation has been treated in Bhattacharya et al. (1983), Gross and Huber-Carol (1992), Gross and Lai (1992) and He and Yang (2003). Regarding random double-truncation, general regression problems have received more attention recently, see e.g. Shen (2013, 2015) and Moreira et al. (2016). Based on some of the key ideas of these works, Frank and Dörre (2017) derived the estimation procedure which is presented here.

We denote the variable, whose distribution is of interest, as Y_i^*, the row vector of covariates as $\mathbf{Z}_i^* = (Z_{i1}^*, \ldots, Z_{ik}^*)$ and the lower and upper truncation variables as U_i^* and $V_i^* = U_i^* + D_i^*$, where D_i^* is a positive variable. Note that we choose to write the upper truncation variable as $V_i^* = U_i^* + D_i^*$ just for later convenience, as technically it is equivalent to use V_i^* in general without the notion of D_i^*. The vector $(Y_i^*, \mathbf{Z}_i^*, U_i^*, D_i^*)$ is observed if and only if $U_i^* \leqslant Y_i^* \leqslant U_i^* + D_i^*$. Their observable counterparts are denoted as Y_i, $\mathbf{Z}_i$, U_i and D_i. In addition, notations without subscript are used to represent corresponding vectors and matrices, e.g. $\mathbf{Y} = (Y_1, \ldots, Y_n)$ and $\mathbf{Z} = (\mathbf{Z}_1^\mathsf{T}, \ldots, \mathbf{Z}_n^\mathsf{T})^\mathsf{T}$. We assume that Y_i^* is the response variable of the linear regression model

$$Y_i^* = \mathbf{Z}_i^* \boldsymbol{\beta} + \varepsilon_i^*,$$

which holds for all units in the latent population before truncation. In the usual sense, $\boldsymbol{\beta}$ denotes the deterministic column vector of regression coefficients and ε_i^* is a random error term. The main goal is to estimate $\boldsymbol{\beta}$. Since the observed values do not represent the latent population's distribution, the conventional estimator $\widehat{\boldsymbol{\beta}} = (\mathbf{Z}^\mathsf{T}\mathbf{Z})^{-1}\mathbf{Z}^\mathsf{T}\mathbf{Y}$ is not valid under double-truncation (see He and Yang 2003). In order to estimate $\boldsymbol{\beta}$ with doubly truncated samples, we utilize a fundamental relation. Note that before truncation,

$$\mathbf{Z}_i^{*\mathsf{T}}Y_i^* = \mathbf{Z}_i^{*\mathsf{T}}\mathbf{Z}_i^* \boldsymbol{\beta} + \mathbf{Z}_i^{*\mathsf{T}}\varepsilon_i^*,$$

and therefore, if $\mathbf{Z}_i^*$ and ε_i^* are independent and $\mathrm{E}(\varepsilon_i^*) = 0$,

$$\mathrm{E}(\mathbf{Z}_i^{*\mathsf{T}}Y_i^*) = \mathrm{E}(\mathbf{Z}_i^{*\mathsf{T}}\mathbf{Z}_i^*)\boldsymbol{\beta} + \mathrm{E}(\mathbf{Z}_i^{*\mathsf{T}}\varepsilon_i^*) = \mathrm{E}(\mathbf{Z}_i^{*\mathsf{T}}\mathbf{Z}_i^*)\boldsymbol{\beta},$$

with respect to the expectations corresponding to the latent population. Thus, if the matrix $\mathrm{E}(\mathbf{Z}_i^{*\mathsf{T}}\mathbf{Z}_i^*)$ is regular,

$$\boldsymbol{\beta} = (\mathrm{E}(\mathbf{Z}_i^{*\mathsf{T}}\mathbf{Z}_i^*))^{-1}\mathrm{E}(\mathbf{Z}_i^{*\mathsf{T}}Y_i^*). \tag{5.1}$$

The conventional maximum likelihood estimator $\widehat{\boldsymbol{\beta}}$ results by substituting these expectations with their empirical estimates, if no truncation is present. However, the empirical distributions are biased under truncation, and thus their true means can not be directly estimated. In fact, when the data are subject to truncation, ε_i^* becomes biased and thus the above reasoning is not valid for the corresponding moments of the observed random variables. Therefore, the crucial step is to estimate the expectations of the latent distributions indirectly using the observed data (see Fig. 5.1). Once this is achieved, the regression coefficients are estimated using Eq. (5.1), i.e. via

$$\widehat{\boldsymbol{\beta}} = (\widehat{\mathrm{E}}(\mathbf{Z}_i^{*\mathsf{T}}\mathbf{Z}_i^*))^{-1}\widehat{\mathrm{E}}(\mathbf{Z}_i^{*\mathsf{T}}Y_i^*).$$

Section 5.2 contains detailed explanations on the model and how estimation of the latent distributions is carried out. In Sect. 5.3, we assess the properties of the resulting

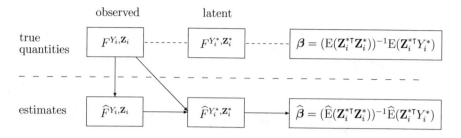

Fig. 5.1 General scheme for estimating the regression coefficients under double-truncation

estimator. It turns out that the proposed estimator of the regression coefficients is consistent and asymptotically normal. For illustration in a practical context, in Sect. 5.4 we apply the method to the German company data, which has been introduced in Chap. 1.

5.2 Model and Method

The primary step is to relate the observed joint distribution of $(Y_i, \mathbf{Z}_i)$ to its latent counterpart. For this, note that if $(Y_i^*, \mathbf{Z}_i^*)$ and (U_i^*, D_i^*), and U_i^* and D_i^* are independent (see assumption (A3) in Sect. 5.3),

$$
\begin{aligned}
F^{Y_i, \mathbf{Z}_i}(y, \mathbf{z}) &= \mathrm{P}\left(Y_i^* \leqslant y, \mathbf{Z}_i^* \leqslant \mathbf{z} \,\middle|\, U_i^* \leqslant Y_i^* \leqslant U_i^* + D_i^*\right) \\
&= \frac{1}{\alpha} \mathrm{P}\left(\{Y_i^* \leqslant y, \mathbf{Z}_i^* \leqslant \mathbf{z}\} \cap \{U_i^* \leqslant Y_i^* \leqslant U_i^* + D_i^*\}\right) \\
&= \frac{1}{\alpha} \int_0^y \int_{-\infty}^{\mathbf{z}} \left\{ \int_0^\infty F^{U_i^*}(u) - F^{U_i^*}(u-d) \, d F^{D_i^*}(d) \right\} \, d F^{Y_i^*, \mathbf{Z}_i^*}(u, \mathbf{w}),
\end{aligned}
$$

and hence

$$
d F^{Y_i^*, \mathbf{Z}_i^*}(y, \mathbf{z}) = \frac{\alpha}{\int_0^\infty F^{U_i^*}(y) - F^{U_i^*}(y-d) \, d F^{D_i^*}(d)} d F^{Y_i, \mathbf{Z}_i}(y, \mathbf{z}). \tag{5.2}
$$

This relation is the key to deal with the unknown joint distribution of $(Y_i^*, \mathbf{Z}_i^*)$. It holds that

$$
\begin{aligned}
\mathrm{E}\left(\mathbf{Z}_{i,l}^* \mathbf{Z}_{i,m}^*\right) &= \int_0^\infty \int_{-\infty}^\infty \mathbf{z}_l \mathbf{z}_m \, d F^{Y_i^*, \mathbf{Z}_i^*}(y, \mathbf{z}) \\
&= \alpha \int_0^\infty \int_{-\infty}^\infty \frac{\mathbf{z}_l \mathbf{z}_m}{\int_0^\infty F^{U_i^*}(y) - F^{U_i^*}(y-d) \, d F^{D_i^*}(d)} \, d F^{Y_i, \mathbf{Z}_i}(y, \mathbf{z}) \tag{5.3}
\end{aligned}
$$

and

$$E\left(Y_i^* \mathbf{Z}_{i,m}^*\right) = \int\limits_0^\infty \int\limits_{-\infty}^\infty y\mathbf{z}_m \, dF^{Y_i^*,\mathbf{Z}_i^*}(y, \mathbf{z})$$

$$= \alpha \int\limits_0^\infty \int\limits_{-\infty}^\infty \frac{y\mathbf{z}_m}{\int_0^\infty F^{U_i^*}(y) - F^{U_i^*}(y-d) \, dF^{D_i^*}(d)} \, dF^{Y_i,\mathbf{Z}_i}(y, \mathbf{z}), \quad (5.4)$$

for $l, m \in \{1, \ldots, k\}$, i.e. the latent moments can be expressed as weighted moments of the observed variables. To establish estimates for $E(\mathbf{Z}_{i,l}^* \mathbf{Z}_{i,m}^*)$ and $E(Y_i^* \mathbf{Z}_{i,m}^*)$, several distribution estimates are necessary. Regarding $F^{Y_i,\mathbf{Z}_i}$, we choose the empirical distribution function $\widehat{F}^{Y_i,\mathbf{Z}_i}(y, \mathbf{z}) := n^{-1} \sum I(Y_i \leqslant y, \mathbf{Z}_i \leqslant \mathbf{z})$, which is consistent with respect to the observed distributions. Discrete non-parametric estimators for F^{U_i} and $F^{U_i+D_i}$ are provided by the NPMLE (see Chap. 4). Specifically, define $\widehat{k}^{(0)} := (1/n, \ldots, 1/n)$ and $\widehat{K}_j^{(t)} := \sum_{i=1}^n \widehat{k}_i^{(t)} I(U_i \leqslant Y_j \leqslant U_i + D_i), t \in \mathbb{N}$. The density estimate of $F^{U_i^*, U_i^*+D_i^*}$ is calculated by iterating

$$\widehat{k}_i^{(t+1)} = \left(\sum_{j=1}^n \frac{I(U_i \leqslant Y_j \leqslant U_i + D_i)}{\widehat{K}_j^{(t)}}\right)^{-1}, \quad i = 1, \ldots, n$$

until reaching t^* such that $\|\widehat{k}^{(t^*)} - \widehat{k}^{(t^*-1)}\| < \epsilon$ for a chosen $\epsilon > 0$. The estimators for the lower, upper and the joint truncation distribution are given by

$$\widehat{F}^{U_i^*}(u) := \sum_{i=1}^n \widehat{k}_i^{(t^*)} I(U_i \leqslant u)$$

$$\widehat{F}^{D_i^*}(d) := \sum_{i=1}^n \widehat{k}_i^{(t^*)} I(D_i \leqslant d)$$

$$\widehat{F}^{U_i^*, U_i^*+D_i^*}(u, v) := \sum_{i=1}^n \widehat{k}_i^{(t^*)} I(U_i \leqslant u, \ U_i + D_i \leqslant v).$$

In the following, let $D_{[1]} \leq D_{[2]} \leq \cdots \leq D_{[n]}$ be the ordered values of $D_1, \ldots, D_n$. Using the established estimator for the truncation distribution, the selection probability α is estimated by

$$\widehat{\alpha} = \left(\int\limits_0^\infty \frac{1}{\int_0^\infty \widehat{F}^{U_i^*}(y) - \widehat{F}^{U_i^*}(y-d) \, d\widehat{F}^{D_i^*}(d)} \, d\widehat{F}^{Y_i,\mathbf{Z}_i}(y, \mathbf{z})\right)^{-1}$$

$$= n \left(\sum_{r=1}^n \frac{1}{\sum_{s=1}^n \left[\widehat{F}^{U_i^*}(Y_r) - \widehat{F}^{U_i^*}(Y_r - D_{[s]})\right] \cdot \widehat{f}_s^{D_i^*}}\right)^{-1},$$

where $\widehat{f}_1^{D_i^*} := \widehat{F}^{D_i^*}(D_{[1]})$ and $\widehat{f}_s^{D_i^*} := \widehat{F}^{D_i^*}(D_{[s]}) - \widehat{F}^{D_i^*}(D_{[s-1]}), s = 2, \ldots, n$. Plugging $\widehat{\alpha}$, $\widehat{F}^{Y_i, Z_i}$, $\widehat{F}^{U_i^*}$ and $\widehat{F}^{D_i^*}$ into Eq. (5.3) yields

$$\widehat{E}\left(Z_{i,l}^* Z_{i,m}^*\right) := \widehat{\alpha} \int_0^\infty \frac{z_l z_m}{\int_0^\infty \widehat{F}^{U_i^*}(y) - \widehat{F}^{U_i^*}(y - d) \, d\widehat{F}^{D_i^*}(d)} \, d\widehat{F}^{Y_i, Z_i}(y, z)$$

$$= \frac{\widehat{\alpha}}{n} \sum_{r=1}^n \frac{Z_{r,l} Z_{r,m}}{\sum_{s=1}^n \left[\widehat{F}^{U_i^*}(Y_r) - \widehat{F}^{U_i^*}(Y_r - D_{[s]})\right] \cdot \widehat{f}_s^{D_i^*}}.$$

The estimated expectation $\widehat{E}(Z_{i,m}^* Y_i^*)$ is defined analogously via Eq. (5.4). Finally, the estimator for β is given by

$$\widehat{\beta} := (\widehat{E}(Z_i^{*\mathsf{T}} Z_i^*))^{-1} \widehat{E}(Z_i^{*\mathsf{T}} Y_i^*), \tag{5.5}$$

if the inverse of $\widehat{E}(Z_i^{*\mathsf{T}} Z_i^*)$ exists. In Appendix F, we provide an implementation of this estimation procedure in R for a simulated dataset.

Note that for calculating $\widehat{\beta}$, the term $\widehat{\alpha}/n$ can be omitted because it gets cancelled out in Eq. (5.5). The variance of ε_i^* is estimated by

$$\widehat{\mathrm{Var}}(\varepsilon_i^*) := \widehat{E}((Y_i^*)^2) - \left[\widehat{E}(Z_i^{*\mathsf{T}} Y_i^*)\right]^\mathsf{T} \widehat{\beta},$$

where $\widehat{E}((Y_i^*)^2)$ is defined analogously to $\widehat{E}(Z_i^{*\mathsf{T}} Z_i^*)$ and $\widehat{E}(Z_i^{*\mathsf{T}} Y_i^*)$ by interchanging z_m with y in Eq. (5.4). In addition, the distribution of ε_i^* can be estimated by

$$\widehat{F}^{\varepsilon_i^*}(x) := \frac{\widehat{\alpha}}{n} \sum_{r=1}^n \frac{I(Y_r - Z_r \widehat{\beta} \le x)}{\sum_{s=1}^n \left[\widehat{F}^{U_i^*}(Y_r) - \widehat{F}^{U_i^*}(Y_r - D_{[s]})\right] \cdot \widehat{f}_s^{D_i^*}}.$$

The coefficient of determination R^2 is a measure to assess the goodness-of-fit of a linear model. The population quantity R^2 is defined as $R^2 = 1 - \mathrm{Var}(\varepsilon^*)/\mathrm{Var}(Y^*)$, which is the proportion of the variation in Y^* that is explained by Z^*. By estimating the two variances, we obtain the estimator of R^2 as

$$\widehat{R}^2 := 1 - \frac{\widehat{\mathrm{Var}}(\varepsilon_i^*)}{\widehat{E}((Y_i^*)^2) - \widehat{E}(Y_i^*)^2}.$$

Up to here, the presented estimates constitute the standard array of quantities for the linear regression model. For obtaining standard errors and thus confidence intervals for the estimated regression coefficients, a bootstrap method is suggested (see Chap. 4 and Moreira and Uña-Álvarez 2010). Specifically, the B bootstrap resamples are defined as *iid* draws from the observed data. For each bootstrap sample $b \in \{1, \ldots, B\}$, the estimate $\widehat{\beta}^{(b)}$ (and the additional quantities) are calculated, thus yielding a pseudo-empirical distribution, based on which standard errors and confidence intervals can be derived.

5.3   Properties of the Estimators

We show consistency and asymptotic normality of $\widehat{\beta}$ by applying the functional delta method. For any given random variable X, define $a_X := \inf\{x \,|\, F^X(x) > 0\}$ and $b_X := \inf\{x \,|\, F^X(x) = 1\}$, so that the support of X is (a_X, b_X). The following conditions are assumed.

(A1) The truncation variables U_i^* and D_i^* are independent and continuous random variables and $P(D_i^* > 0) = 1$.

(A2) Every component of $(\varepsilon_i^*, \mathbf{Z}_i^*)$ is square-integrable.

(A3) Y_i^* and (U_i^*, D_i^*) are quasi-independent (see Chap. 1 for a definition of quasi-independence).

(A4) $E(\varepsilon_i^*) = 0$ and $\text{Cov}(\mathbf{Z}_i^*, \varepsilon_i^*) = 0$.

(A5) $\alpha := P(U_i^* \le Y_i^* \le U_i^* + D_i^*) > 0$.

(A6) $a_{F^{U_i^*}} \le a_{F^{Y_i^*}} \le a_{F^{U_i^*+D_i^*}}$ and $b_{F^{U_i^*}} \le b_{F^{Y_i^*}} \le b_{F^{U_i^*+D_i^*}}$.

From a practical point of view, most of these assumptions are not critical. In many applications, (A1) and (A4) are fulfilled because the truncation variables U_i^* and D_i^* often represent time which can usually be thought of as being continuous and $D_i^* > 0$ naturally. Regarding D_i^*, many applications in the literature on random double-truncation (see e.g. Kalbfleisch and Lawless 1989; Moreira and Uña-Álvarez 2010 and also Sect. 5.4) in fact deal with a known constant D_i^*, which further simplifies calculations. Square-integrability of covariates and error terms, as required by (A2), is a classical assumption and not an issue for real data sets. In contrast, quasi-independence as defined in Tsai (1990) of response and truncation variables is not obviously fulfilled. If the sampling mechanism does not imply this assumption, it is recommended to use appropriate tests (e.g. Efron and Petrosian 1999; Martin and Betensky 2005; Emura and Wang 2010; Shen 2011) in order to check (A3). Assumption (A6) is important to ensure that the whole support of the response variable can be observed and hence the distribution of interest is identifiable (see He and Yang 2003; Shen 2010 and Chap. 4). For non-parametric methods under random double-truncation, there is no workaround for this assumption. Note that (A5) is implied by (A6) and only stated for more convenient reasoning in the remainder.

In the setting of Shen (2010), $F^{Y_i^*}$ is also non-parametrically estimated, say by $\breve{F}^{Y_i^*}$. Shen (2010) proves uniform consistency of $\breve{F}^{Y_i^*}$ for fixed $[a_{F^{Y_i^*}}, t] \subset [0, \infty]$, $t \in (a_{F^{Y_i^*}}, b_{F^{Y_i^*}})$ under the following additional assumptions:

(B1) $[a_{F^{Y_i^*}}, t]$ is such that $F^{Y_i^*}(v) - F^{Y_i^*}(u-) > \delta > 0$ for $[u, v] \subset [a_{F^{Y_i^*}}, t]$.

(B2) $\displaystyle\int_{a_{F^{Y_i^*}}}^{t} \frac{d F^{Y_i^*}(y)}{F^{U_i^*, U_i^*+D_i^*}(y, \infty) - F^{U_i^*, U_i^*+D_i^*}(y, y)} < \infty.$

(B3) $\dfrac{d F^{U_i^*, U_i^*+D_i^*}(y, \infty) - d F^{U_i^*, U_i^*+D_i^*}(y, y)}{d F^{Y_i^*}(y)}$ is uniformly bounded on $[a_{F^{Y_i^*}}, t]$.

The uniform consistency of $\check{F}^{Y_i^*}$ implies the uniform consistency of $\widehat{F}^{U_i^*,U_i^*+D_i^*}$. Assumption (B1) ensures that $F^{Y_i^*}(v) - F^{Y_i^*}(u-)$ is uniformly bounded away from zero. Condition (B2) holds if $a_{F^{U_i^*}} < a_{F^{U_i^*}}$ and $a_{F^{Y_i^*}} \leq a_{F^{U_i^*,U_i^*+D_i^*}}$. Therefore (A6) and $a_{F^{U_i^*}} \neq a_{F^{Y_i^*}}$ imply (B2). The last assumption (B3) holds if the density of $(U_i^*, U_i^* + D_i^*)$ is bounded from above and the density of Y_i^* is positive on $[a_{F^{Y_i^*}}, t]$. Considering real data sets, assumptions (B1) and (B3) are not critical. In applications, for (B1) and (B3) it only has to be assumed that the distribution of Y_i^* has no inner intervals where the density is zero.

In order to prove the consistency and asymptotic normality of $\widehat{\beta}$ under the assumptions (A1)–(A6) and (B1)–(B3), it will be shown first that $\widehat{E}(Z_i^{*\mathsf{T}}Z_i^*)$ and $\widehat{E}(Z_i^{*\mathsf{T}}Y_i^*)$ are consistent and asymptotically normal. This is carried out with a mapping theorem for weak convergence and the central limit theorem. Afterwards, the multivariate delta method is applied to complete the proof. The consistency of the other estimators follows analogously. For the sake of clarity, the generalized mapping theorem is restated first (see Billingsley 1968, p. 34).

Lemma 5.1 *Let h_n and h be measurable mappings from Ω to Ω', P_n and P be probability measures on Ω and E be the set of x such that $h_n(x_n) \to h(x)$ fails to hold for some sequence $\{x_n\}$ approaching x. If $P_n \to P$ and $P(E) = 0$, then $P_n h_n^{-1} \to P h^{-1}$.*

To avoid ambiguities, let f be a real function on Ω'. Then f is integrable with respect to Ph^{-1} if and only if $f \circ h$ is integrable with respect to P and, by definition, it holds that (Billingsley 1968, p. 223)

$$\int f(h(x))dP(x) = \int f(x')dPh^{-1}(x').$$

Theorem 5.1 *Under the model assumptions (A1)–(A6) and (B1)–(B3), it holds that*

$$\widehat{E}(Z_i^{*\mathsf{T}}Z_i^*) \xrightarrow{\mathcal{P}} E(Z_i^{*\mathsf{T}}Z_i^*)$$
$$\widehat{E}(Z_i^{*\mathsf{T}}Y_i^*) \xrightarrow{\mathcal{P}} E(Z_i^{*\mathsf{T}}Y_i^*),$$

where $\xrightarrow{\mathcal{P}}$ denotes convergence in probability.

Proof The proof consists of two steps, each using the generalized mapping theorem. In both steps, $\Omega' := \mathbb{R}_+$ whereas h_n, h, Ω, E, P_n and P differ. Let $y \in [a_{F^{Y_i^*}}, b_{F^{Y_i^*}}]$ be fixed, then

$$\int_0^\infty \widehat{F}^{U_i^*}(y) - \widehat{F}^{U_i^*}(y-x) d\widehat{F}^{D_i^*}(x) = \int_0^\infty h_n^{(1)}(x) d P_n^{(1)}(x)$$

$$\xrightarrow{n\to\infty} \int_0^\infty h^{(1)}(x) d P^{(1)}(x)$$

$$= \int_0^\infty F^{U_i^*}(y) - F^{U_i^*}(y-x) d F^{D_i^*}(x),$$

where $\Omega^{(1)} := \mathbb{R}_{\geq 0}$, $h^{(1)}(x) := F^{U_i^*}(y) - F^{U_i^*}(y-x)$, $h_n^{(1)}(x) := \widehat{F}^{U_i^*}(y) - \widehat{F}^{U_i^*}(y-x)$, $P^{(1)} := F^{D_i^*}$ and $P_n^{(1)} := \widehat{F}^{D_i^*}$. Because of the uniform consistency of $F^{U_i^*}$, it holds that $E^{(1)} = \emptyset$. For $l, m \in \{1, \dots, k\}$, let

$$h_n^{(2)}(y, \mathbf{z}) := \frac{\mathbf{z}_l \mathbf{z}_m}{\int_0^\infty \widehat{F}^{U_i^*}(y) - \widehat{F}^{U_i^*}(y-x) d\widehat{F}^{D_i^*}(x)}$$

$$h^{(2)}(y, \mathbf{z}) := \frac{\mathbf{z}_l \mathbf{z}_m}{\int_0^\infty F^{U_i^*}(y) - F^{U_i^*}(y-x) d F^{D_i^*}(x)},$$

where $\Omega^{(2)} := \mathbb{R}^1 \times \mathbb{R}^k$. Assumption (A5) is necessary to ensure that $\int_0^\infty F^{U_i^*}(y) - F^{U_i^*}(y-x) d F^{D_i^*}(x) > 0$. The same inequality is true for the related estimator if there is at least one observation. Therefore, the continuous mapping theorem with the function $x \mapsto 1/x$ implies $h_n^{(2)}(y, \mathbf{z}) \xrightarrow{n\to\infty} h^{(2)}(y, \mathbf{z})$. In addition, $E^{(2)} = (-\infty, a_{F^{U_i^*}}) \times \emptyset$ which is a null set as long as assumption (A6) holds. Choosing $P_n^{(2)} := \widehat{F}^{Y_i, \mathbf{Z}_i}$ and $P^{(2)} := \widehat{F}^{Y_i, \mathbf{Z}_i}$ allows for the second use of the mapping theorem. To complete the proof, the estimator $\widehat{\alpha}$ needs to be consistent. However, just consider the special case of $h_n^{(2)}(y, \mathbf{z})$ where $z_l z_m = 1$ to show that $1/\widehat{\alpha} \to 1/\alpha$. Then, the application of the continuous mapping theorem implies the consistency of $\widehat{\alpha}$. Again, $\widehat{\alpha}$ can not be zero if there is at least one observation. Finally, Slutsky's theorem completes the proof, i.e.

$$\widehat{\mathbb{E}}(\mathbf{Z}_i^{*\top}\mathbf{Z}_i^*)_{l,m} = \widehat{\alpha} \cdot \int_0^\infty \frac{\mathbf{z}_l \mathbf{z}_m}{\int_0^\infty \widehat{F}^{U_i^*}(y) - \widehat{F}^{U_i^*}(y-x) d\widehat{F}^{D_i^*}(x)} d\widehat{F}^{Y_i, \mathbf{Z}_i}(y, \mathbf{z})$$

$$\xrightarrow{n\to\infty} \alpha \cdot \int_0^\infty \frac{z_l z_m}{\int_0^\infty F^{U_i^*}(y) - F^{U_i^*}(y-x) d F^{D_i^*}(x)} d F^{Y_i, \mathbf{Z}_i}(y, \mathbf{z})$$

$$= \mathbb{E}(\mathbf{Z}_i^{*\top}\mathbf{Z}_i^*)_{l,m}.$$

The proof of

$$\widehat{\mathbb{E}}(\mathbf{Z}_i^{*\top} Y_i^*) \xrightarrow{\mathcal{P}} \mathbb{E}(\mathbf{Z}_i^{*\top} Y_i^*)$$

follows analogously by interchanging $\mathbf{z}_m$ and y. $\square$

Corollary 5.1 *Assume that* $\det(\widehat{E}(\mathbf{Z}_i^{*\mathsf{T}}\mathbf{Z}_i^*)) \neq 0$ *almost surely asymptotically. Then the estimator*

$$\widehat{\boldsymbol{\beta}} := (\widehat{E}(\mathbf{Z}_i^{*\mathsf{T}}\mathbf{Z}_i^*))^{-1}\widehat{E}(\mathbf{Z}_i^{*\mathsf{T}}Y_i^*)$$

is consistent, i.e. $\widehat{\boldsymbol{\beta}} \xrightarrow{P} \boldsymbol{\beta}$.

Proof As long as the inverse of $\widehat{E}(\mathbf{Z}_i^{*\mathsf{T}}\mathbf{Z}_i^*)$ exists, $\widehat{\boldsymbol{\beta}}$ is a composition of continuous functions with the components of $\widehat{E}(\mathbf{Z}_i^{*\mathsf{T}}\mathbf{Z}_i^*)$ and $\widehat{E}(\mathbf{Z}_i^{*\mathsf{T}}Y_i^*)$ as arguments. The continuous mapping theorem implies the weak consistency of $\widehat{\boldsymbol{\beta}}$, which is equivalent to $\widehat{\boldsymbol{\beta}} \xrightarrow{P} \boldsymbol{\beta}$, since $\boldsymbol{\beta}$ is constant (see Theorem 2.3 and Theorem 2.7 in van der Vaart 1998).   □

Corollary 5.2 *It holds that*

(i) $\widehat{\mathrm{Var}}(\varepsilon_i^*) \xrightarrow{P} \mathrm{Var}(\varepsilon_i^*)$
(ii) $\widehat{F}^{\varepsilon_i^*} \xrightarrow{P} F^{\varepsilon_i^*}$
(iii) $\widehat{R}^2 \xrightarrow{P} R^2$

Proof The properties easily follow from Theorem 5.1.   □

Theorem 5.2 *The estimators* $\widehat{E}(\mathbf{Z}_i^{*\mathsf{T}}\mathbf{Z}_i^*)_{l,m}$ *and* $\widehat{E}(\mathbf{Z}_i^{*\mathsf{T}}Y_i^*)_m$ *are asymptotically normal for all* $l, m \in \{1, \ldots, k\}$.

Proof The main idea is to show that the estimated means can be asymptotically expressed as a mean of *iid* random variables. For details, see Theorem 2 in Frank and Dörre (2017).   □

Corollary 5.3 *Assume that* $\det(\widehat{E}(\mathbf{Z}_i^{*\mathsf{T}}\mathbf{Z}_i^*)) \neq 0$ *almost surely asymptotically. Then* $\widehat{\boldsymbol{\beta}}$ *is asymptotically normal and consistent.*

Proof The assertion follows directly from Theorem 5.2 and the multivariate delta method (see van der Vaart 1998).   □

5.4 Application

We estimate a linear regression model for a subset of the insolvency dataset, considering all companies which were founded in the German federal state Hesse. The restriction to this state is chosen in order to avoid possible heterogeneity between different states and regions. The main interest is the companies' lifetime until insolvency, measured in days. The sample contains $n = 400$ companies which became insolvent between September 1, 2013 and March 31, 2014. Thus the constant observation period consists of $D_i^* \equiv 211$ days. We define Y_i^* as the age at insolvency of the i-th company and U_i^* as the age at September 1, 2013. Therefore, the i-th company

Fig. 5.2 Three examples for foundation (black bullet) and insolvency (white bullet) of observed (solid) and truncated (dashed) companies

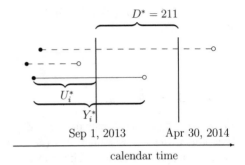

is observed if and only if $U_i^* \le Y_i^* \le U_i^* + D_i^*$. Figure 5.2 illustrates the truncation mechanism.

The data set constitutes a special case for the truncation model, because D^* has only probability mass in 211. In this case, the calculation of the weights is slightly easier because

$$\int_0^\infty \widehat{F}^{U^*}(y) - \widehat{F}^{U^*}(y-u)\, d\widehat{F}^{D^*}(u) = \widehat{F}^{U^*}(y) - \widehat{F}^{U^*}(y - D^*).$$

Due to the sampling mechanism, assumption (A3) is reasonable. Note that (A6) is fulfilled because

$$a_{F^{U^*}} = 0 < a_{F^{Y^*}} = 1 \ < a_{F^{U^*+D^*}} = 214$$
$$b_{F^{U^*}} = \infty \le b_{F^{Y^*}} = \infty \le b_{F^{U^*+D^*}} = \infty.$$

Here $a_{F^{Y_i^*}} = 1$ because a company is assumed to survive at least for one day. This also implies the validity of assumption (B2). Every observation has the following 8 dummy covariates:

$Z_{i,1}$ constant 1 for all observations
$Z_{i,2}$ equal to 1 for limited liability companies, limited partnerships or hybrids
$Z_{i,3}$ equal to 1 for entrepreneurial companies with limited liability
$Z_{i,4}$ equal to 1 for companies in the manufacturing sector
$Z_{i,5}$ equal to 1 for companies in the building sector
$Z_{i,6}$ equal to 1 for companies in the commerce sector
$Z_{i,7}$ equal to 1 for companies in the maintenance sector
$Z_{i,8}$ equal to 1 for companies in the car repair sector.

Determining the estimates and bootstrapping standard errors for confidence intervals yields Table 5.1. Note that the standard errors are bootstrapped with 1000 resamples.

We obtained $R^2 = 0.054$. Hence, 5.4% of the variation in companies' lifetime is explained by the eight covariates. Even though the model has not particularly high

Table 5.1 Estimation results with confidence intervals and standard errors

		90% confidence intervals		
		Estimate	Lower bound	Upper bound
Intercept	$\widehat{\beta}_1$	3923.4	2494	5351
Limited liability/partnership	$\widehat{\beta}_2$	96.1	−1273	1465
Entrepreneurial company	$\widehat{\beta}_3$	−3073.7	−4457	−1689
Manufacturing sector	$\widehat{\beta}_4$	−717.5	−1667	232
Building sector	$\widehat{\beta}_5$	1536.2	275	2796
Commerce sector	$\widehat{\beta}_6$	218.0	−702	1140
Maintenance sector	$\widehat{\beta}_7$	−25.8	−968	944
Car repair sector	$\widehat{\beta}_8$	636.2	−513	1785
			Estimated standard error	
Selection probability	$\widehat{\alpha}$	0.0101	0.0012	
Population size	$\widehat{N}$	39,598	4192	
Error variance	$\widehat{\mathrm{Var}}(\varepsilon^*)$	12,381,425	1,476,544	
Coefficient of determination	$\widehat{R}^2$	0.054	0.040	

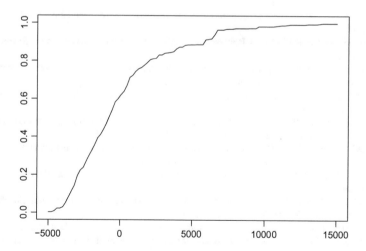

Fig. 5.3 Estimated distribution function of ε^*

goodness-of-fit, it is noted that $\widehat{\beta}_1$, $\widehat{\beta}_3$ and $\widehat{\beta}_5$ are significantly different from zero (at 90%). Therefore, entrepreneurial companies seem to exhibit a higher insolvency risk compared to other company forms. This is not surprising because an entrepreneurial company often has relatively low capital and, according to national law, may become a limited liability company once it has accumulated enough share capital. Regarding the different sectors, the building sector $(\widehat{\beta_5})$ has a lower insolvency risk compared to other sectors. The remaining sectors are clearly insignificant, and hence seem to have no effect on the age at insolvency in this model.

Apparently, the confidence intervals for the estimated coefficients are quite large. One reason for this is the relatively small sample size $n = 400$. The estimated error distribution function $\widehat{F}^{\varepsilon^*}$ (see Fig. 5.3) possesses an asymmetric shape. In addition, the corresponding standard deviation of the error terms $\widehat{\mathrm{Var}}(\varepsilon^*)^{0.5} \approx 3519$ indicates that the model lacks further covariates, preferably having a metric scale.

References

Bhattacharya PK, Chernoff H, Yang SS (1983) Nonparametric estimation of the slope of a truncated regression. Ann Stat 11(2):505–514

Billingsley P (1968) Convergence of probability measures. Wiley series in probability and statistics. Wiley, New York

Efron B, Petrosian V (1999) Nonparametric methods for doubly truncated data. J Am Stat Assoc 94(447):824–834

Emura T, Konno Y, Michimae H (2015) Statistical inference based on the nonparametric maximum likelihood estimator under double-truncation. Lifetime Data Anal 21:397–418

Emura T, Wang W (2010) Testing quasi-independence for truncation data. J Multivar Anal 101:223–239

Frank G, Dörre A (2017) Linear regression with randomly double-truncated data. South Afr Stat J 51(1):1–18

Gross ST, Huber-Carol C (1992) Regression models for truncated survival data. Scand J Stat 19(3):193–213

Gross ST, Lai TL (1996) Nonparametric estimation and regression analysis with left-truncated and right-censored data. J Am Stat Assoc 91(435):1166–1180

He S, Yang GL (2003) Estimation of regression parameters with left truncated data. J Stat Plan Inference 117(1):99–122

Kalbfleisch J, Lawless JF (1989) Inference based on retrospective ascertainment: an analysis of the data on transfusion-related aids. J Am Stat Assoc 84(406):360–372

Martin EC, Betensky RA (2005) Testing quasi-independence of failure and truncation times via conditional Kendall's tau. J Am Stat Assoc 100:484–492

Moreira C, Uña-Álvarez J (2010) Bootstrapping the NPMLE for doubly truncated data. J Nonparametric Stat 22(5):567–583

Moreira C, Uña-Álvarez J, Meira-Machado L (2016) Nonparametric regression with doubly truncated data. Comput Stat Data Anal 93:294–307

Shen P-S (2010) Nonparametric analysis of doubly truncated data. Ann Inst Stat Math 62:835–853

Shen P-S (2011) Testing quasi-independence for doubly truncated data. J Nonparametric Stat 23(3):753–761

Shen P-S (2013) Regression analysis of interval censored and doubly truncated data with linear transformation models. Comput Stat 28:581–596

Shen P-S (2015) Median regression model with doubly truncated data. J Appl Stat 42:360–370

Tsai W-Y (1990) Testing the assumption of independence of truncation time and failure time. Biometrika 77:169–177

van der Vaart A (1998) Asymptotic statistics. Cambridge University Press, United Kingdom

Appendix A
Formula of the SE for the NPMLE

Let $\hat{\mathbf{f}} = (\hat{f}_1, \ldots, \hat{f}_n)^{\mathrm{T}}$ be the NPMLE computed on the masses at the ordered values $y_{(1)} < \cdots < y_{(n)}$. Especially, $\hat{f}_n$ is the mass corresponding to the largest observation $y_{(n)} = \max_i(y_i)$. Let J be an $n \times n$ matrix whose (i, j) component is $J_{ij} = I(u_i \leq y_j \leq v_i)$. Also, let $\hat{F}_i = \sum_{m=1}^n \hat{f}_m J_{im}$ be the estimated masses on $[u_i, v_i]$ for $i = 1, \ldots, n$. Then, it follows that $\hat{\mathbf{F}} = J\hat{\mathbf{f}}$, where $\hat{\mathbf{F}} = (\hat{F}_1, \ldots, \hat{F}_n)^{\mathrm{T}}$.

As in Emura et al. (2015), we define $SE\{\hat{F}(t)\} = \sqrt{\hat{V}\{\hat{F}(t)\}}$, where the estimator of the asymptotic variance is

$$\hat{V}\{\hat{F}(t)\} = \mathbf{W}_t^{\mathrm{T}}\left[D\left\{\mathrm{diag}\left(\frac{1}{\hat{\mathbf{f}}^2}\right) - J^{\mathrm{T}}\mathrm{diag}\left(\frac{1}{\hat{\mathbf{F}}^2}\right)J\right\}D^{\mathrm{T}}\right]^{-1}\mathbf{W}_t,$$

where $\mathbf{W}_t = (I(y_{(1)} \leq t) - I(y_{(n)} \leq t), \ldots, I(y_{(n-1)} \leq t) - I(y_{(n)} \leq t))^{\mathrm{T}}$, $D = [I_{n-1}\vdots{-}\mathbf{1}_{n-1}]$, where I_{n-1} is the identity matrix of dimension $n-1$, $\mathbf{1}_n = (1, \ldots, 1)^{\mathrm{T}}$ is n-vector of ones, and $\mathrm{diag}(\mathbf{a})$ is a diagonal matrix with the diagonal elements $\mathbf{a}$. The estimator of the asymptotic covariance is

$$\hat{C}ov\{\hat{F}(s), \hat{F}(t)\} = \mathbf{W}_s^{\mathrm{T}}\left[D\left\{\mathrm{diag}\left(\frac{1}{\hat{\mathbf{f}}^2}\right) - J^{\mathrm{T}}\mathrm{diag}\left(\frac{1}{\hat{\mathbf{F}}^2}\right)J\right\}D^{\mathrm{T}}\right]^{-1}\mathbf{W}_t.$$

Reference

Emura T, Konno Y, Michimae H (2015) Statistical inference based on the non-parametric maximum likelihood estimator under double-truncation. Lifetime Data Anal 21(3): 397–418

Appendix B
Score Function and Hessian Matrix
in a Two-Parameter Model

The score function and Hessian matrix are the first- and second-order derivatives of the log-likelihood function that is defined by

$$
\ell(\boldsymbol{\eta}) = \sum_{i=1}^{n} \eta_1 y_i + \sum_{i=1}^{n} \eta_2 y_i^2 + \frac{n\eta_1^2}{4\eta_2} + \frac{n}{2} \log(-\eta_2) - \frac{n}{2} \log(\pi)
$$
$$
- \sum_{i=1}^{n} \log \left\{ \Phi\left(\frac{v_i + \frac{\eta_1}{2\eta_2}}{\sqrt{\frac{-1}{2\eta_2}}} \right) - \Phi\left(\frac{u_i + \frac{\eta_1}{2\eta_2}}{\sqrt{\frac{-1}{2\eta_2}}} \right) \right\},
$$

where the parameter space is $\Theta = \{(\eta_1, \eta_2) : \eta_1 \in \mathbb{R}, \eta_2 < 0\}$.

Let $\phi(.)$ be the density of $N(0, 1)$. Following the notations of Cohen (1991, p. 32), we let

$$
H_{i1}(\eta_1, \eta_2) \equiv \frac{\phi\left(\frac{v_i + \frac{\eta_1}{2\eta_2}}{\sqrt{\frac{-1}{2\eta_2}}} \right)}{\Phi\left(\frac{v_i + \frac{\eta_1}{2\eta_2}}{\sqrt{\frac{-1}{2\eta_2}}} \right) - \Phi\left(\frac{u_i + \frac{\eta_1}{2\eta_2}}{\sqrt{\frac{-1}{2\eta_2}}} \right)}, \quad H_{i2}(\eta_1, \eta_2) \equiv \frac{\phi\left(\frac{u_i + \frac{\eta_1}{2\eta_2}}{\sqrt{\frac{-1}{2\eta_2}}} \right)}{\Phi\left(\frac{v_i + \frac{\eta_1}{2\eta_2}}{\sqrt{\frac{-1}{2\eta_2}}} \right) - \Phi\left(\frac{u_i + \frac{\eta_1}{2\eta_2}}{\sqrt{\frac{-1}{2\eta_2}}} \right)},
$$

which are analogous to the hazard functions in the presence of double-truncation (Sankaran and Sunoj 2004). The derivatives of these hazard functions are explicitly written e.g. as.

© The Author(s), under exclusive license to Springer Nature Singapore Pte Ltd. 2019
A. Dörre and T. Emura, *Analysis of Doubly Truncated Data*, JSS Research
Series in Statistics, https://doi.org/10.1007/978-981-13-6241-5

$$\frac{\partial}{\partial \eta_1} H_{i1} = \sqrt{\frac{-1}{2\eta_2}} H_{i1} \left[\frac{v_i + \frac{\eta_1}{2\eta_2}}{\sqrt{\frac{-1}{2\eta_2}}} + H_{i1} - H_{i2} \right],$$

$$\frac{\partial}{\partial \eta_1} H_{i2} = \sqrt{\frac{-1}{2\eta_2}} H_{i2} \left[\frac{u_i + \frac{\eta_1}{2\eta_2}}{\sqrt{\frac{-1}{2\eta_2}}} + H_{i2} - H_{i1} \right].$$

The first derivatives of the log-likelihood (score functions) are

$$\frac{\partial}{\partial \eta_1} \ell(\boldsymbol{\eta}) = \sum_{i=1}^{n} y_i + \frac{n\eta_1}{2\eta_2} + \frac{1}{\sqrt{-2\eta_2}} \sum_{i=1}^{n} \{ H_{i1}(\eta_1, \eta_2) - H_{i2}(\eta_1, \eta_2) \},$$

$$\frac{\partial}{\partial \eta_2} \ell(\boldsymbol{\eta}) = \sum_{i=1}^{n} y_i^2 - \frac{n\eta_1^2}{4\eta_2^2} + \frac{n}{2\eta_2} - \sum_{i=1}^{n} \left\{ H_{i1}(\eta_1, \eta_2) \cdot \left(\frac{-v_i}{\sqrt{-2\eta_2}} - \eta_1 \frac{\sqrt{-2\eta_2}}{4\eta_2^2} \right) \right\}$$

$$+ \sum_{i=1}^{n} \left\{ H_{i2}(\eta_1, \eta_2) \cdot \left(\frac{-u_i}{\sqrt{-2\eta_2}} - \eta_1 \frac{\sqrt{-2\eta_2}}{4\eta_2^2} \right) \right\}.$$

The second-order derivatives of the log-likelihood are

$$\frac{\partial^2}{\partial \eta_1^2} \ell(\boldsymbol{\eta}) = \frac{n}{2\eta_2} - \frac{1}{2\eta_2} \sum_{i=1}^{n} \left\{ H_{i1}(\eta_1, \eta_2) \left(\frac{v_i + \frac{\eta_1}{2\eta_2}}{\sqrt{\frac{-1}{2\eta_2}}} \right) - H_{i2}(\eta_1, \eta_2) \left(\frac{u_i + \frac{\eta_1}{2\eta_2}}{\sqrt{\frac{-1}{2\eta_2}}} \right) \right\}$$

$$- \frac{1}{2\eta_2} \sum_{i=1}^{n} \{ H_{i1}(\eta_1, \eta_2) - H_{i2}(\eta_1, \eta_2) \}^2,$$

$$\frac{\partial^2}{\partial \eta_2^2} \ell(\boldsymbol{\eta}) = + \frac{n\eta_1^2}{2\eta_2^3} - \frac{n}{2\eta_2^2}$$

$$+ \sum_{i=1}^{n} \left\{ H_{i1}(\eta_1, \eta_2) \left(\frac{-v_i}{\sqrt{-2\eta_2}} - \eta_1 \frac{\sqrt{-2\eta_2}}{4\eta_2^2} \right) - H_{i2}(\eta_1, \eta_2) \left(\frac{-u_i}{\sqrt{-2\eta_2}} - \eta_1 \frac{\sqrt{-2\eta_2}}{4\eta_2^2} \right) \right\}^2$$

$$+ \sum_{i=1}^{n} H_{i1}(\eta_1, \eta_2) \left[\left(\frac{v_i + \frac{\eta_1}{2\eta_2}}{\sqrt{\frac{-1}{2\eta_2}}} \right) \left(\frac{-v_i}{\sqrt{-2\eta_2}} - \eta_1 \frac{\sqrt{-2\eta_2}}{4\eta_2^2} \right)^2 - \left(\frac{-v_i}{\sqrt{(-2\eta_2)^3}} - \frac{3\eta_1}{\sqrt{(-2\eta_2)^5}} \right) \right]$$

$$- \sum_{i=1}^{n} H_{i2}(\eta_1, \eta_2) \left[\left(\frac{u_i + \frac{\eta_1}{2\eta_2}}{\sqrt{\frac{-1}{2\eta_2}}} \right) \left(\frac{-u_i}{\sqrt{-2\eta_2}} - \eta_1 \frac{\sqrt{-2\eta_2}}{4\eta_2^2} \right)^2 - \left(\frac{-u_i}{\sqrt{(-2\eta_2)^3}} - \frac{3\eta_1}{\sqrt{(-2\eta_2)^5}} \right) \right],$$

$$\frac{\partial^2}{\partial \eta_1 \partial \eta_2} \ell(\boldsymbol{\eta}) = -\frac{n\eta_1}{2\eta_2^2} + (-2\eta_2)^{\frac{-3}{2}} \sum_{i=1}^{n} \{H_{i1}(\eta_1,\eta_2) - H_{i2}(\eta_1,\eta_2)\}$$

$$-\frac{1}{\sqrt{-2\eta_2}} \sum_{i=1}^{n} \left[H_{i1}(\eta_1,\eta_2) \left(\frac{v_i + \frac{\eta_1}{2\eta_2}}{\sqrt{\frac{-1}{2\eta_2}}} \right) \left\{ \frac{-v_i}{\sqrt{-2\eta_2}} - (-2\eta_2)^{\frac{-3}{2}}\eta_1 \right\} \right]$$

$$+\frac{1}{\sqrt{-2\eta_2}} \sum_{i=1}^{n} \left[H_{i2}(\eta_1,\eta_2) \left(\frac{u_i + \frac{\eta_1}{2\eta_2}}{\sqrt{\frac{-1}{2\eta_2}}} \right) \left\{ \frac{-u_i}{\sqrt{-2\eta_2}} - (-2\eta_2)^{\frac{-3}{2}}\eta_1 \right\} \right]$$

$$-\frac{1}{\sqrt{-2\eta_2}} \sum_{i=1}^{n} \left[\{H_{i1}(\eta_1,\eta_2) - H_{i2}(\eta_1,\eta_2)\} \left[\begin{array}{c} H_{i1}(\eta_1,\eta_2)\left\{ \frac{-v_i}{\sqrt{-2\eta_2}} - (-2\eta_2)^{\frac{-3}{2}}\eta_1 \right\} \\ -H_{i2}(\eta_1,\eta_2)\left\{ \frac{-u_i}{\sqrt{-2\eta_2}} - (-2\eta_2)^{\frac{-3}{2}}\eta_1 \right\} \end{array} \right] \right].$$

References

Cohen AC (1991) Truncated and Censored Samples. Marcel Dekker, New York

Sankaran PG, Sunoj SM (2004) Identification of models using failure rate and mean residual life of doubly truncated random variables. Stat Pap 45:97–109

Appendix C
R Codes for the Analysis of Childhood Cancer Data

Below, we provide our R codes for analyzing the childhood cancer data (Chap. 2). The codes require the users to install the R package *double.truncation* (Emura et al. 2019) . Since we do not have a copyright to reproduce the original data, we created a toy dataset that mimics the original dataset of Moreira and de Uña-Álvarez (2010). Consequently, the R codes below produce slightly different numerical results from those of Chap. 2. To produce the numerical results of Chap. 2, please replace the toy dataset by the original data available in Table 8 of Moreira and de Uña-Álvarez (2010).

© The Author(s), under exclusive license to Springer Nature Singapore Pte Ltd. 2019
A. Dörre and T. Emura, *Analysis of Doubly Truncated Data*, JSS Research
Series in Statistics, https://doi.org/10.1007/978-981-13-6241-5

```
library(double.truncation) ## install the R package

## Toy data similar to Table 8 of Moreira and de Uña-Álvarez (2010)
y.trunc=c(5,10,15,40,85,90,95,100,105,120,130,145,160,165,170,200,205,220,230,250,250,275,280,290,295,
    300,310,315,320,325,330,335,345,350,360,365,370,375,380,385,395,420,435,450,455,460,465,470,475,480,
    505,510,515,520,525,530,540,545,560,575,580,585,590,595,600,615,620,625,635,640,655,665,670,675,680,
    700,710,715,735,740,750,760,770,775,785,790,810,820,835,840,845,850,855,860,870,875,890,895,
    900,910,915,940,945,965,970,975,985,1000,1005,1010,1015,1020,1025,1030,1035,1040,1045,1050,1050,1055,
    1055,1060,1065,1070,1080,1095,1100,1105,1110,1130,1155,1165,1175,1180,1185,1195,
    1205,1220,1225,1230,1240,1245,1250,1255,1265,1300,1320,1325,1335,1345,1360,1370,1375,1400,1410,1420,
    1450,1465,1485,1490,1495,1500,1505,1515,1520,1520,1520,1530,1550,1555,1560,1575,
    1600,1600,1610,1620,1680,1690,1690,1695,1725,1730,1740,1750,1755,1790,1795,
    1800,1805,1810,1815,1825,1860,1880,1885,1890,1960,2025,2030,2040,2050,2060,2065,
    2105,2140,2145,2165,2170,2173,2173,2180,2195,2210,2235,2250,2275,2280,2285,2290,2295,
    2320,2330,2340,2345,2350,2355,2365,2370,2415,2425,2435,2440,2445,2460,2475,2480,
    2505,2525,2565,2570,2581,2585,2585,2600,2609,2613,2647,2649,2658,2660,2675,2695,
    2700,2705,2730,2735,2735,2790,2800,2805,2815,2940,2950,2960,2980,2985,2990,2995,
    3050,3070,3075,3085,3105,3125,3130,3155,3260,3260,3265,3270,3275,3300,3335,3340,3345,3365,3375,3385,
    3420,3445,3465,3475,3490,3515,3545,3560,3605,3640,3670,3685,3685,3690,3710,3775,3815,3830,3860,3875,
    3940,3955,3990,4005,4005,4025,4040,4080,4080,4080,4145,4150,4205,4240,4245,4250,4275,4280,4350,4385,
    4410,4420,4425,4445,4445,4450,4475,4475,4480,4495,4515,4520,4520,4525,4550,4555,4560,4570,4580,4585,
    4600,4600,4625,4670,4675,4730,4745,4750,4790,4790,4795,4800,4830,4845,4850,4855,4885,4890,4895,4895,
    4905,4910,4920,4955,4960,4985,4985,4990,5045,5055,5055,5060,5070,5075,5145,5150,5155,5175,5190,5195,
    5210,5220,5235,5255,5275,5295,5315,5340,5350,5375,5380,5435,5435,5440,5440,5450,5455,5475)

u.trunc=c(-1645,-25,-532,-1505,-690,-1235,-785,-260,-110,-120,-705,-1620,-330,-45,20,-1505,-535,-535,-250,-875,
    -1155,-60,-935,-650,-40,-1010,-585,-690,-320,220,60,-1280,-900,110,-510,-590,-415,-535,-625,-45,335,-785,285,
    -315,-1145,330,-1165,-700,460,-1160,-1235,-480,-400,160,315,-45,25,-885,350,395,10,-1140,-250,-515,-860,-850,
```

```
-870,505,-185,60,-875,-275,-980,465,135,-750,100,-30,-390,585,475,545,40,200,-790,455,-225,-850,-690,-230,545,
-610,-715,-175,260,570,255,380,-710,90,765,-125,-790,955,240,695,-435,190,60,-140,-620,-550,680,-355,700,
-605,645,-365,290,225,725,670,855,-245,900,545,-410,440,810,-180,515,645,170,790,-590,800,-435,785,645,960,
-240,510,-435,40,520,-495,40,290,515,875,1180,485,1165,825,-50,905,1115,250,785,975,545,525,21,1305,55,
410,345,640,-50,945,-115,-65,195,20,450,615,770,-20,1355,140,-30,55,680,910,1360,85,1370,125,645,1355,915,
580,1585,380,970,1550,1625,260,1060,2040,380,1790,1300,935,690,900,1890,1075,775,1475,845,740,2130,
1750,1340,2195,1945,1095,1500,1690,1930,1710,670,765,920,1655,1940,580,2325,980,1890,860,985,1885,1745,
2150,2325,1670,1835,1870,1910,1310,2555,2145,905,1695,2220,1005,1575,1585,2460,2195,2700,1945,1615,
2155,1705,2335,1310,2405,1930,2820,2460,2565,1590,1390,2410,2445,1245,1965,1495,2615,2340,1905,1485,
1880,1710,1700,1835,2140,2175,2115,2390,1845,2125,3000,3320,1910,3090,2440,2125,2320,3335,3335,2605,
1830,3335,2665,3365,2260,3175,3355,2340,2955,2085,2070,2110,2780,3300,3710,2370,3520,3640,3540,2430,
3145,3835,3845,3490,4025,2501,4145,3945,3980,3755,2895,2890,2750,3500,3690,4115,3715,2955,2840,2680,
4264,3933,3950,4423,3303,3788,4250,4399,2972,3853,3204,3455,3645,4235,4235,4540,4275,4405,3025,3800,
2965,4790,4425,3760,4010,3825,3055,3970,4485,4070,4680,3715,3925,3140,4620,4190,4105,4230,4715,4240,
4240,4525,3870,4115,4395,4280,4770,3380,4940,4735,4750,3730,4465,4380,4095,3990,5255,5125,4375,4310,
4915,3645,4245,3815,3670,5345,3825,530,3875,3780,4990)

v.trunc=u.trunc+1825 ### upper truncation limit
n=length(y.trunc)

#### MLE under seven different models ####
PMLE.SEF1.positive(u.trunc, y.trunc, v.trunc,epsilon = 1e-05)
PMLE.SEF1.negative(u.trunc, y.trunc, v.trunc,epsilon = 1e-05)
PMLE.SEF1.free(u.trunc, y.trunc, v.trunc,epsilon = 1e-05)
PMLE.SEF2.negative(u.trunc, y.trunc, v.trunc,epsilon = 1e-05)
PMLE.SEF3.positive(u.trunc, y.trunc, v.trunc,epsilon = 1e-05)
PMLE.SEF3.negative(u.trunc, y.trunc, v.trunc,epsilon = 1e-05)
PMLE.SEF3.free(u.trunc, y.trunc, v.trunc,epsilon = 1e-05)


#### NPMLE ####
S.NP=1- NPMLE(u.trunc, y.trunc, v.trunc,epsilon=1e-08)$F ### survival probabilities
y.o=sort(y.trunc)
plot(y.o,S.NP,xlab="age (in days)",ylab="Survival probability", type="S",col=1,lwd=2)

#### MLE under the SEF 1 model ####
SEF1.free=PMLE.SEF1.free(u.trunc, y.trunc, v.trunc,epsilon = 1e-05)
eta_hat=SEF1.free$eta1
tau1=min(y.trunc)
tau2=max(y.trunc)
```

```
S=( exp(eta_hat*tau2)-exp(eta_hat*y.o) )/( exp(eta_hat*tau2)-exp(eta_hat*tau1) )
points(y.o,S,col=2,type="l",cex=2,lwd=2)


dS1=( tau2*exp(eta_hat*tau2)-y.o*exp(eta_hat*y.o) )/( exp(eta_hat*tau2)-exp(eta_hat*tau1) )
dS2=( tau2*exp(eta_hat*tau2)-tau1*exp(eta_hat*y.o) )/( exp(eta_hat*tau2)-exp(eta_hat*tau1) )
dS=dS1-S*dS2
SE1.free=sqrt( -dS^2/SEF1.free$Hessian    )
points(y.o,S+1.96*SE1.free,col=2,type="l",lty="dotted")
points(y.o,S-1.96*SE1.free,col=2,type="l",lty="dotted")


legend(2000,1,legend=c("One-parameter model","Pointwise 95%CI","NPMLE"),
       ,col=c("red","red","black"),lty=c(1,2,1),lwd=c(2,1,2))
```

References

Emura T, Hu YH, Huang CY (2019) double.truncation: analysis of doubly-truncated data, CRAN
Moreira C, de Uña-Álvarez J (2010) Bootstrapping the NPMLE for doubly truncated data.
    J Nonparametr Stat 22:567–583

Appendix D
R Code for Bayesian Analysis of Doubly Truncated Data

In this appendix, we provide an R code for analyzing simulated doubly truncated data with a fully parametric Bayesian model (Chap. 3).

```
#-------------------------------------------------------------
# Script for Bayesian Analysis of Doubly Truncated Data
#-------------------------------------------------------------

require(mcmc)

#tv is the vector of time points that define the birth interval
#e.g., tv = c(0, 6, 8) defines two birth periods (0, 6) and (6, 8)
tv = c(0, 6, 8)

#selection interval (tL, tR) in which units are sampled
tL = 8
tR = 10

#vector of the birth process parameters
lambdak = c(1000, 1000)

#parameter for the lifetime distribution (Exp distribution as example)
theta = 1.0

#settings for Metropolis algorithm
#(NMCMC: output size, thinning: number of thinned replications)
NMCMC = 5000
thinning = 20

#step size for numerical integration
intd = 0.01

#step size for numerical derivatives
h = 0.001

#coverage level and non-coverage level for interval estimation
CIlevel = 0.95
CInlevel = 1-CIlevel

#determination of period variables
m = length(tv) - 1
sk = tv[1:m]
tk = tv[2:(m+1)]
```

```
#——————————————————————————————————
# Functions for Implementation of the Metropolis Algorithm
#——————————————————————————————————

#selection probability for k-th birth period (under Exp distribution)
pk <- function(k, theta){
   z1 = exp(-theta*tL) - exp(-theta*tR)
   z2 = exp(theta*tk[k]) - exp(theta*sk[k])
   z3 = (tk[k]-sk[k])*theta
   z = z1*z2/z3
   return(z)
}

#marginal loglikelihood function
loglike_marg <- function(theta){
   S = -Inf
   if (min(theta)>0){
      S = n*log(theta) - theta*Sy
      for (k in 1:m){
         p = pk(k, theta)
         S = S - (nk[k]+1)*log(p)
      }
   }
   return(S)
}

#setting for the log prior density, return(0) for uniform prior
log_prior <- function(prms){
   return(0)
}

#posterior log density
posterior_log_density_marg <- function(prms){
   S = loglike_marg(prms) + log_prior(prms)
   return(S)
}

#names of the parameters
prms_names = c()
for (k in 1:m){
   prms_names = c(prms_names, paste('lambda', k, sep=''))
}
prms_names = c(prms_names, 'theta')

#cumulative birth intensities for each birth period
Lambdak = lambdak*(tk-sk)
```

```
#————————————————————————————————————————————————
# Generation of Simulated Dataset
#————————————————————————————————————————————————

#simulation of random births in the latent population
bb = c()
Nk = 1:m
for (k in 1:m){
  Nk[k] = rpois(1, Lambdak[k])
  bb = c(bb, runif(Nk[k], sk[k], tk[k]))
}
N = sum(Nk)

#random lifetimes in the latent population
yy = rexp(N, theta)

#determining the selected units after truncation
sam = (bb+yy>=tL) & (bb+yy <= tR)
b = bb[sam]
y = yy[sam]
n = length(b)

y = y[order(b)]
b = sort(b)

#calculating the number of observations for each birth period
nk = rep(0, m)
for (k in 1:m){
  nk[k] = sum(I(sk[k] <= b)*I(b <= tk[k]))
}
print(nk)


#histogram of sampled births
hist(b, main='Histogram␣of␣observed␣births', xlab='')


#————————————————————————————————————————————————
# MCMC Simulation of the marginal posterior density
#————————————————————————————————————————————————

#initializing parameter value (as first guess)
prms0 = 1/mean(y)
nprms = 1

#determination of (part of) the sufficient statistics
Sy = sum(y)

#initiale estimate of a reasonal proposal standard deviation
sd_proposal = 1/(sqrt(n*prms0))
```

```
#first simulation of the posterior distribution
zmarg1 = metrop(posterior_log_density_marg, initial=prms0, nbatch=1000,
                blen = 1, nspac = 3, scale = sd_proposal)$batch
plot(zmarg1[,1], typ='l', ylab='theta')

#update of MCMC settings for the Metropolis algorithm
prms0 = colMeans(zmarg1)
sd_proposal = sd(zmarg1)

#second simulation of the posterior distribution
zmarg = metrop(posterior_log_density_marg, initial=prms0, nbatch=NMCMC,
               blen = 1, nspac = thinning, scale = sd_proposal)$batch
plot(zmarg[,1], typ='l', ylab='theta')

#autocorrelation plot (autocorrelation should be small for Lag>0)
acf(zmarg[,1], main='Autocorrelation_of_output_sequence')

#conditional simulation of lambdak based on zmarg
lambdak_simM = matrix(0, NMCMC, m)
for (j in 1:NMCMC){
  thetaj = zmarg[j,]
  for (k in 1:m){
    lambdak_simM[j,k] = rgamma(1, nk[k]+1, (tk[k]-sk[k])*pk(k, thetaj))
  }
}




#──────────────────────────────────────────────
# Simulation Results
#──────────────────────────────────────────────

#posterior mean for the lifetime parameter(s)
theta_est = colMeans(zmarg)
print(theta_est)

#posterior mean for the birth process parameters
lambdak_est = colMeans(lambdak_simM)
print(lambdak_est)

#Ey: estimate of the mean lifetime
Ey = mean(1/zmarg)
print(Ey)
```

```r
#approximating the pointwise confidence band
yseq = seq(0.01, max(tv), 0.05)
CBd = c()
CBp = c()
CBh = c()
for (yp in yseq){
  dv = dexp(yp, zmarg)
  CBd = rbind(CBd, quantile(dv, c(CInlevel/2, 1-CInlevel/2)))
  pv = pexp(yp, zmarg)
  CBp = rbind(CBp, quantile(pv, c(CInlevel/2, 1-CInlevel/2)))
  hv = dv/(1-pv)
  CBh = rbind(CBh, quantile(hv, c(CInlevel/2, 1-CInlevel/2)))
}


#plot of the density and confidence band
plot(yseq, dexp(yseq, theta_est), main='Estimated_Density_Function',
     xlab='lifetime_(years)', ylab='', typ='l', ylim=c(0,max(CBd)))
lines(yseq, CBd[,1], lty=2)
lines(yseq, CBd[,2], lty=2)


#plot of the distribution function and confidence band
plot(yseq, pexp(yseq, theta_est), main='Estimated_Distribution_Function',
     xlab='lifetime_(years)', ylab='', typ='l', ylim=c(0,max(CBp)))
lines(yseq, CBp[,1], lty=2)
lines(yseq, CBp[,2], lty=2)


#plot of the hazard function and confidence band
hgamma = dexp(yseq, theta_est)/(1-pexp(yseq, theta_est))
plot(yseq, hgamma, main='Estimated_Hazard_Function',
     xlab='lifetime_(years)', ylab='', typ='l', ylim=c(0,max(CBh)))
lines(yseq, CBh[,1], lty=2)
lines(yseq, CBh[,2], lty=2)


#joining the simulated values
z = cbind(lambdak_simM, zmarg)
colnames(z) = prms_names

#Bayesian point estimate of the parameters
prms_est = colMeans(z)
print(prms_est)

#posterior variance as estimate of the point estimate variance
V_est = var(z)
print(V_est)
```

```
nprms = length(prms_est)
#estimation of confidence intervals (posterior quantiles)
CIB = matrix(0, nprms, 2)
for (j in 1:nprms){
  CIB[j,] = quantile(z[,j], c(CInlevel/2, 1−CInlevel/2))
}
rownames(CIB) = prms_names
colnames(CIB) = c('lower', 'upper')
print(CIB)

#plot of the birth intensity including confidence bounds
Q = CIB
plot(c(sk[1], tk[1]), c(prms_est[1], prms_est[1]),
     xlim=c(sk[1], tR), ylim=c(0,1.1*max(Q)), typ='l',
     ylab='Estimated_Intensity_of_Birth_Process', xlab='calendar_time')
lines(c(sk[1], tk[1]), c(Q[1,1], Q[1,1]), lty=2)
lines(c(sk[1], tk[1]), c(Q[1,2], Q[1,2]), lty=2)
for (k in 2:m){
  lines(c(sk[k], tk[k]), c(prms_est[k], prms_est[k]))
  for (j in 1:2){
    lines(c(sk[k], tk[k]), c(Q[k,j], Q[k,j]), lty=2)
  }
}
```

Appendix E
R Code for Non-parametric Analysis
of Doubly Truncated Data

In this appendix, we provide an R code for analyzing the Equipment-S dataset with the NPMLE (Chap. 4).

```
#————————————————————————————————————————
# Script for Nonparametric Analysis of the Equipment-S dataset
#————————————————————————————————————————
library(double.truncation)

u = c(4,0.7,4.7,0.6,6.7,1.2,0.6,7.2,2.2,7.7,5.2,5.2,1.8,5.9,2.7,1.7,2.8,
      5.1,4.4,7.8,8.9,5.8,9,10.3,6.3,0.2,1.4,3.2,0.5,8.5,5.6,7.4,5.7,8.9,
      8.1,10.7,10.9,10.9,3.9,5,3.3,6.9,7.9,7.8,14.2,8,1.2,12,0.4,9.4,8.9,
      7.9,12.8,5.8,3.5,7.5,1.2,4.8,3.7,3.1,6.9,16,4.3,6.2,2.7,7.6,6,8.2,
      6.3,12.5,8.4,11.4,10.8,6.1,12.8,15.2,4.7,4.8,4.6,15,8.8,9.7,17.1,3.5,
      16.5,9.3,11.2,10.5,4.8,11.7,8.7,15.7,14.2,10.1,9.8,16.5,18.2,14.5,
      4.5,15,12.8,16.5,9.8,17,6.2,6.8,11.2,10.7,17.6,9.3,9.8,10.2,6.6,15.9,
      8.9,7.9,10.3,7.6,18.4,13,7.7,17.8,16.6,13.2,7.2,15.3,14.5,12.8,16.3,
      14.5,18.6,9,17.9,12.9,15.5,16.8,11.9,17.1,17.2,13.8,10.7,11.3,17.8,
      18.2,18.2,12.8,18.9,18.8,18.8,12,13.5,17,17.7,18.3,16.8,17.9,18.5,16.7,
      16.8,18.6,18.9,17.7,18.6)
y = c(4.7,6,6.4,6.5,7.5,7.6,7.7,8,8.1,8.3,8.4,8.5,8.6,8.7,8.9,9.2,9.3,9.4,
      9.6,9.7,9.8,10.3,10.4,10.7,10.8,10.8,10.9,11.1,11.1,11.2,11.7,11.7,
      11.8,11.8,11.9,12.1,12.7,13.2,13.3,13.4,13.8,13.9,14,14.3,14.3,14.4,
      14.5,14.5,14.6,14.8,15.2,15.2,15.4,15.5,15.6,15.7,15.7,15.8,16.1,16.2,
      16.2,16.3,16.3,16.5,16.5,16.8,16.9,16.9,17.1,17.2,17.2,17.2,17.2,17.5,
      17.6,17.6,17.6,17.7,17.8,17.8,18.2,18.3,18.3,18.4,18.6,18.6,18.7,18.8,
      18.8,18.9,19.2,19.3,19.4,19.6,19.6,19.9,20,20.1,20.2,20.2,20.3,20.3,
      20.4,20.5,20.5,20.5,20.7,20.8,20.8,20.9,20.9,21.7,22,22,22.2,22.3,
      22.3,22.3,22.4,22.5,22.6,22.7,22.7,22.8,23,23.5,23.7,23.8,23.8,23.9,
      23.9,23.9,24,24.1,24.1,24.3,24.4,24.4,24.5,25,25,25.3,25.8,25.8,26.1,
      26.9,27.6,27.6,27.7,27.7,28.1,29.5,29.8,29.8,30,30.5,30.7,30.9,32.2,
      32.3,33.4,33.6,34.5)
v = c(20,16.7,20.7,16.6,22.7,17.2,16.6,23.2,18.2,23.7,21.2,21.2,17.8,21.9,
      18.7,17.7,18.8,21.1,20.4,23.8,24.9,21.8,25,26.3,22.3,16.2,17.4,19.2,
      16.5,24.5,21.6,23.4,21.7,24.9,24.1,26.7,26.9,26.9,19.9,21,19.3,22.9,
      23.9,23.8,30.2,24,17.2,28,16.4,25.4,24.9,23.9,28.8,21.8,19.5,23.5,17.2,
      20.8,19.7,19.1,22.9,32,20.3,22.2,18.7,23.6,22,24.2,22.3,28.5,24.4,27.4,
      26.8,22.1,28.8,31.2,20.7,20.8,20.6,31,24.8,25.7,33.1,19.5,32.5,25.3,
      27.2,26.5,20.8,27.7,24.7,31.7,30.2,26.1,25.8,32.5,34.2,30.5,20.5,31,
      28.8,32.5,25.8,33,22.2,22.8,27.2,26.7,33.6,25.3,25.8,26.2,22.6,31.9,
      24.9,23.9,26.3,23.6,34.4,29,23.7,33.8,32.6,29.2,23.2,31.3,30.5,28.8,
      32.3,30.5,34.6,25,33.9,28.9,31.5,32.8,27.9,33.1,33.2,29.8,26.7,27.3,
      33.8,34.2,34.2,28.8,34.9,34.8,34.8,28,29.5,33,33.7,34.3,32.8,33.9,34.5,
      32.7,32.8,34.6,34.9,33.7,34.6)

result = NPMLE(u, y, v)



#plot of the distribution function including confidence intervals
Fest = result$F
SE = result$SE
plot(y, Fest, typ='l', xlim=c(0, 35), xlab='Lifetime', ylab='',
     main='Estimated Lifetime Distribution')
lines(y, Fest - 1.96*SE, lty=2)
lines(y, Fest + 1.96*SE, lty=2)
```

Appendix F
R Code for Linear Regression Under Random Double Truncation

In this appendix, we provide an R code for analyzing simulated doubly truncated data with a linear regression model (Chap. 5).

© The Author(s), under exclusive license to Springer Nature Singapore Pte Ltd. 2019   107
A. Dörre and T. Emura, *Analysis of Doubly Truncated Data*, JSS Research
Series in Statistics, https://doi.org/10.1007/978-981-13-6241-5

```r
#-----------------------------------------------
# Script for Nonparametric Analysis of Doubly Truncated Data
#-----------------------------------------------

#size of latent population
N = 300

#parameters for the linear regression model (single regressor)
beta = c(-3, 5)
sigma = 1


#-----------------------------------------------
# Generation of Simulated Dataset
#-----------------------------------------------

#random regressors (constant 1 and uniform on (0,3))
Z = cbind(rep(1, N), runif(N, 0, 3))

#random error terms
eps = rnorm(N, 0, sigma)

#random lifetimes in the latent population
yy = Z %*% beta + eps

#random truncation times
uu = runif(N, -5, 3)
vv = runif(N, 7, 14)

#determining the selected units after truncation
sam = (uu <= yy) & (yy <= vv)
y = yy[sam]
u = uu[sam]
v = vv[sam]
z = Z[sam, ]
n = length(y)


#calculation of the NPMLE
library(double.truncation)
result = NPMLE(u, y, v)
```

```r
#indicator matrix J for determining the density k
J = matrix(0, n, n)
for (m in 1:n){
  for (i in 1:n){
    J[m, i] = as.numeric((u[m] <= y[i]) && (y[i] <= v[m]))
  }
}


fest = result$f
Fest = J %*% fest
SFestInv = (sum(1/Fest))^(-1)
kest = rep(0, n)
for (i in 1:n){
  kest[i] = SFestInv/Fest[i]
}


#-----------------------------------------------------------
# Implementation of the Linear Regression Estimate
#-----------------------------------------------------------

#estimated latent distribution functions
FU <- function(t){return(sum(kest[u<=t]))}
FD <- function(t){return(sum(kest[d<=t]))}

#estimation of moment matrices
q = length(beta)
EZZ = matrix(0, q, q)
EZY = matrix(0, q, 1)
d = v-u
ds = sort(d)

S = 0
for (i in 1:n){
  Ri = 0
  for (j in 1:n){
    if (j>=2){
      fD = FD(ds[j]) - FD(ds[j-1])
    }else{fD = FD(ds[1])}
    FUdiff = FU(y[i]) - FU(y[i] - ds[j])
    Ri = Ri + FUdiff*fD
  }
  S = S + 1/Ri
  for (l in 1:q){
    EZY[l, 1] = EZY[l, 1] + y[i]*z[i, l]/Ri
    for (m in 1:q){
      EZZ[l, m] = EZZ[l, m] + z[i, l]*z[i, m]/Ri
    }
  }
}
```

```
alpha_est = n/S
EZZ = EZZ*alpha_est/n
EZY = EZY*alpha_est/n

beta_est = solve(EZZ) %*% EZY
print(beta_est)
```

Index

© The Author(s), under exclusive license to Springer Nature Singapore Pte Ltd. 2019
A. Dörre and T. Emura, *Analysis of Doubly Truncated Data*, JSS Research
Series in Statistics, https://doi.org/10.1007/978-981-13-6241-5

Printed in the United States
By Bookmasters